The Parents' Guide
to Cochlear Implants

The Parents' Guide
to Cochlear Implants

Patricia M. Chute
Mary Ellen Nevins

Gallaudet University Press
Washington, D.C.

Gallaudet University Press
Washington, DC 20002

© 2002 by Gallaudet University
All rights reserved. Published 2002
Printed in Canada

http://gupress.gallaudet.edu

Library of Congress Cataloging-in-Publication Data

Chute, Patricia M.
    The parents' guide to cochlear implants / Patricia M. Chute, Mary Ellen Nevins.
        p. cm.
    Includes bibliographical references and index.
    ISBN 1-56368-129-3 (alk. paper)
        1. Cochlear implants. 2. Hearing impaired children–Rehabilitation. 3.
    Deaf–Rehabilitation. I. Nevins, Mary Ellen. II. Title.

    RF305.C487 2002
    617.8'82—dc21

                                                            2002072390

Book design: David Alcorn, Alcorn Publication Design
Cover photograph: John T. Consoli
Cover models: Tammy Gavins and Destinee Gavins
Figures 3.1, 3.2, 3.5, and 5.1 are courtesy of Cochlear Corporation, figures 3.3 and
3.6 are courtesy of Advanced Bionics Corporation, and figures 3.4 and 3.7 are
courtesy of Med El Corporation.

♾ The paper used in this publication meets the minimum requirements of American
National Standard for Information Sciences—Permanence of Paper for Printed Library
Materials, ANSI Z39.48–1984.

Contents

We dedicate this book to our own parents

Louis and Marie Molinelli
and
Donald and Shelia Nevins

Our partners in parenting
Bob Chute, Sr.
and
Warren O'Leary

And all the parents lost in the World Trade Center attack on
September 11, 2001

Acknowledgments

A number of individuals contributed in a variety of ways to the writing of this book. We would like to acknowledge the constant support and friendship of Amy Popp who has always come to the rescue during our writing frenzies. Her organizational knowledge, computer skills, and sensitivity to our outbursts of frustration have been much appreciated through the years. We would also like to recognize the hard work of Nichole Czarnecki for compiling the parent responses for the chapter in which parents speak for themselves. Simon C. Parisier, M.D., the surgeon with the vision and perspective that has always allowed us to go beyond the traditional models of patient care, also deserves our heartfelt recognition. In addition, the Children's Hearing Institute, Inc., has provided us with continual support for all our professional endeavors. We thank the Board of Directors of this organization. Similarly, we acknowledge the three manufacturers, Cochlear Corporation, Advanced Bionics Corporation, and Med El Corporation for their constant presence in the profession. Finally, we gratefully acknowledge the support of our colleagues at Mercy College and Kean University as we reached beyond our campuses to share our thoughts and experiences with the broader learning community.

Introduction

Initiating the process of cochlear implantation is a complex task. It combines the hard work of gathering information with the difficulty of making a lifetime decision for a child. Parents wishing to explore this technology need information and support. This book is a resource for parents trying to decide if a cochlear implant is right for their child. It answers many of the questions that parents have, and poses and answers some that they may not have considered. This book is written with the parent's perspective in mind and attempts to present a balanced view of implantation: the process, procedure, and performance results.

Chapter 1 outlines steps for beginning the process, highlighting important factors to consider when choosing an implant center. When parents have a choice in determining which center to select, they should assess numerous characteristics about the center before making their decision. These characteristics are detailed to help parents understand the complexities of center selection. A list of questions that parents can ask is also provided.

Chapter 2 explores the candidacy evaluation, a critical point of entry into the process. Evaluation of children for implantation should be considered within the perspective of the whole child. This whole child perspective sets the stage for understanding performance outcomes after implantation.

Chapter 3 includes an unbiased review of the various implant technologies available, thereby allowing parents to compare and contrast the different implant systems. Issues related to internal components, external components, and accessories are presented so that parents can be satisfied with the device that has been selected. Chapter 4 follows up with a discussion of the surgical procedures and other pre- and post-surgical concerns of parents. Useful tips for the practical realities of the hospital stay and the implant procedure are outlined. Since this is a stressful time for most parents, the more information that is available, the less the parent is caught off guard by unanticipated events.

Initial switch-on, post-implant issues, and the responsibilities of the parents in managing their child's equipment after implantation are reviewed in chapter 5. This is a time in which there is often a great deal of excitement and anticipation, so it is important for parents to have realistic expectations about the initial switch-on and the immediate post-implant period.

In chapter 6, parents learn about strategies that can be used in the home to foster good listening behaviors. This chapter provides parents with an outline to begin the process of helping their youngster develop auditory skills. The role the parent plays in supporting the school and therapy cannot be overstated.

Chapter 7 explores the role of the implant in light of the variety of communication options that are available to children with hearing loss. This chapter establishes that the implant is able to coexist with a variety of communication strategies as long as there is sufficient auditory input and opportunity to use spoken language. No one methodology is required for a child with an implant, nor can any methodology guarantee a particular result for any child.

Chapter 8 addresses the issue of school choice, especially for deaf children who use cochlear implants. With the trends in education changing rapidly in today's society, it is important that parents understand the services that each placement type does and does not provide.

Performance outcomes of the cochlear implant relative to the whole child are outlined in chapter 9, and the candidacy issues outlined in chapter 2 are revisited. Performance can then be viewed from the perspective of the child's skills and abilities at the start of the implant process and how they contribute to ultimate benefit. The notions of implant "success" and "failure" are addressed in a frank and open manner.

Chapter 10 details the evolution of cochlear implants in the context of Deaf culture and considers how cochlear implant users can move comfortably between the hearing and deaf worlds. This may be the first published attempt to look at the achievements that are possible when the Deaf community and the cochlear implant community work together. Indeed, the current generation of implant recipients may serve as "ambassadors" between the deaf and hearing worlds.

The final chapter recognizes that it is helpful for parents to share their own experiences with those who are just beginning the process. Thus, chapter 11 includes a section in which parents reflect upon their own journey through the implant process. The chapter concludes with an essay on parenting entitled "The Millennial Parent." This section reminds parents that they will still face numerous parenting issues that are separate from those that arise from having a child with a cochlear implant.

Chapter 1

Beginning the Process

The moment parents begin to consider cochlear implantation for their child, they embark on a journey. The more knowledge parents have, the better they will recognize that this journey does not simply begin and end with surgery. Rather, it consists of several stages, including the periods of initial information gathering, pre-implant evaluation, surgery, immediate post-implantation events, and long-term monitoring. The process itself starts when the parents ask the question: Can our child benefit from a cochlear implant? The answer to the question will vary from family to family.

Parents who choose an implant for their child are making a commitment, either fully or partially, to integrate that child into the hearing world. That commitment is the overriding reason that parents select implants. In some cases, the hearing world begins with the family. In other cases, the hearing world lies outside the family door. How parents include a deaf child into the family varies. Hearing parents want to communicate with their deaf children in the language of the immediate and extended family. A cochlear implant can often help achieve this goal. Additionally, access to the larger hearing community is made possible through implant technology, although choosing a cochlear implant does not necessarily imply that a parent refuses to accept the child's deafness. Parents have a variety of options at their disposal to help a child identify with his or her deaf side. They may choose any number of ways to foster the child's growth as a deaf individual and as a child with a cochlear implant.

Deaf parents of deaf children also want to communicate with their children in the language of the immediate and extended family. When this language is American Sign Language (ASL), a visual language, a cochlear implant is not necessary. If access to the hearing world is valued as a means to more opportunity, then, in some instances, deaf parents may consider a cochlear implant.

Regardless of the weight that is placed on connection to the hearing world, a family must make a commitment to support the auditory and speech needs of the child receiving the implant. If this commitment is not made from the beginning, the choice of implantation is doomed.

The initial information gathering stage is a critical point for many parents since it will drive the continuation of the entire process. It is important, therefore, that this stage be as comprehensive as possible. This will enable parents to make an informed decision about whether or not to pursue implantation for their child.

Information Gathering

The more knowledge parents have about cochlear implants, the more power they have in making decisions. In today's society, knowledge is power. Gaining this knowledge can sometimes feel like a full-time job. Information about cochlear implants is available from so many sources that parents can feel overwhelmed very quickly. Sometimes parents are so confused by all the information that they may stop trying to make sense of it and decide against the technology. Some might simply give up and rely on someone else's input to make decisions. Should this happen, parents open themselves up to disappointment when they have not participated actively in the process.

The amount of information that any one parent requires to make decisions is very individualized. Some parents will seek only a basic understanding about the implant and the process.

Other parents will explore more in-depth information about how the implant works, what the candidacy criteria for implantation are, what the implant will do, and what kind of commitment and support is needed to make the process successful. A large amount of information is available in booklet form published by a variety of sources, including the manufacturers, implant centers, national and international organizations, and parent groups. These materials may include terminology that is new to parents; without additional guidance, parents may misinterpret some information and draw incorrect conclusions about the implant. It is critical, therefore, for parents to supplement their reading by interviewing knowledgeable professionals who are experienced in implantation. As with any other decision parents make for their child, they should never rely on a single source for information.

Contacting the Implant Center

If a parent decides to continue the process, the next step might be to identify an implant center. Parents may find out about an implant center from their doctor, audiologist, other parents, a television program or newspaper article, teachers at school, or even by contacting the manufacturers. In less-populated parts of the country, parents may find only one implant center. However, in large urban areas, parents may have a choice of centers. When possible, they should investigate the services that each center provides, particularly the services specifically for children, before making their decision. There are a number of basic characteristics that should be present in any implant center that services children; these are crucial for parents to consider.

Characteristics of a Good Pediatric Cochlear Implant Center

In contrast to an adult cochlear implant program staffed by a single implant surgeon and an audiologist, a pediatric cochlear implant facility demands the presence of a multidisciplinary implant team. In addition to the surgeon, team members should include audiologists and speech/language pathologists who are experienced in working with deaf and hard of hearing children. Centers with a strong educational orientation will have a teacher of deaf children as an active member of the team or available on a consultant basis. Other professionals on the team might include a psychologist and/or a social worker. While pediatric cochlear implant experience is preferred; in some portions of the country, this may not be possible.

The choice of an implant center may be influenced by the distance parents must travel, the number of implant systems available, the amount of educational services provided, and the availability of reimbursement by their insurance company. It is also important to determine the center's orientation to the cultural, linguistic, and social needs of the family. Finally, determining the service delivery model offered by the facility may also help parents to select one that suits their needs.

Distance to the Center

An experienced pediatric cochlear implant center may be located hundreds of miles and several hours away from a family's home. Transporting a child (and sometimes siblings) to a distant center may be difficult for families already stressed by the demands of parenting a child with a hearing loss. Consequently, a newly established implant center with less-experienced personnel located closer to home may be an attractive alternative. Parents may choose the closer implant center after investigating available services and ensuring that it can fulfill their child's basic needs.

With respect to the cochlear implant center itself, the services provided (i.e., audiological, speech/language, and medical-surgical) may not be located in one place. Parents may need to meet with the professionals responsible for providing services at a variety of locations. This may be cumbersome for parents with several children who accompany them on their visits to the center. It is important to be aware of this situation before arrival at the implant facility and plan for the management of the day accordingly.

Implant Systems

Parents must know whether the center they are considering provides implants from more than one manufacturer. In some cases, facilities may only dispense one type of implant. Even if this is the case, an informed consumer should be knowledgeable about other systems. Parents should at least know what they are getting and what they are not. They may also wish to find out if the facility provides backup equipment on an immediate or overnight basis in case of equipment breakdown.

Since properly setting a cochlear implant is so crucial to a child's overall performance, it is important that the audiologist be skilled in working with children. Parents should ask about the experience of the clinician who sets the device as well as the schedule for periodic adjustments. Resetting the device will require regular visits to the center, especially during the first year. Some larger centers may even provide this service at the child's school.

Providing Educational Services

Based on the knowledge that children with cochlear implants spend a considerable portion of their waking hours in schools and classrooms, it is important that the implant center team believes in communicating with local school professionals. Some facilities employ a teacher of deaf children as either a full-time team member or a consultant. This individual may be responsible for tasks such as initiating contact with the child's school before the implant surgery, providing information and professional development to school personnel after implantation, and serving as a liaison between the medical and educational facilities on an ongoing basis.

Language and Cultural Issues

The philosophy of an implant center towards the presence of a second language in the home, whether it is sign language or another spoken language, may also be a determining factor in center selection. Some implant teams believe that using sign language limits the degree of benefit that can be achieved from the implant. For this reason, they will not recommend children for implantation unless parents agree to eliminate the use of sign language altogether. This requirement may not be acceptable to parents who find communication with their deaf child eased through the use of sign.

Parents who use a language in the home other than English may wish to investigate the cochlear implant team's attitude toward it. The cochlear implant center should provide translators for parents with limited English proficiency for all meetings with the team. Parents should ask if written materials about cochlear implants are available in their primary language so they can review the information with other family members once they are at home. Obviously, if an implant team member is fluent in the language of the child's home, parents will be drawn to this center.

Choosing the Implant Center

Parents will want to think about the above factors and how each affects their own family situation to determine which ones are the most important to them. Some parents are fortunate to have several well-established cochlear implant centers nearby. If this is the case, parents may wish to meet with the various team members to decide if the center personnel and the family are a good match. Other parents may not have as many options. Nonetheless, it is important to speak with someone via telephone, e-mail, or in person to determine if the desired characteristics of a comprehensive implant center are present.

Unfortunately, given the present state of health care, parents may not have the luxury of choosing an implant center. Sometimes insurance companies make this decision for parents. Although parents can appeal the decision under special circumstances, the insurance system has become less flexible in recent years. If the insurance carrier's choice is different from the parents', the process may begin under a cloud of disappointment.

After selecting an implant center, parents may choose to discuss other issues with implant center staff members at a preliminary meeting. Frequently, the implant center will give parents names of other families who have been through the process already. Families may be matched for the age of the child, ethnic background, geographical location, or communication methodology. In some cases, parents will first make an appointment to meet with the implant surgeon to discuss many of their questions. It is likely that the surgeon will address the medical and surgical issues and leave the discussion regarding actual candidacy and post-implant habilitation for the appropriate implant center team members.

Planning Questions for Implant Center Personnel

When parents move from *thinking* about getting an implant to actually *pursuing* an implant for their child, there are still more questions to ask to ensure that their final decision regarding implantation is an informed one. Answers to these questions may vary somewhat from center to center; the following questions and general responses are offered as a guideline for parents. These include

- How does the implant work?
- What type of evaluation is needed to determine if a child is a candidate?
- What are the general benefits and risks of surgery?
- What are the educational/therapeutic needs of children with implants?
- What are the long-term outcomes?
- What are the time and financial obligations of the parents?
- How do the cochlear implant and Deaf culture coexist?

Answers to these questions may vary somewhat from center to center; the following general responses are offered as a guideline for parents.

How does the implant work?

In order to understand how an implant functions, it is important to understand normal hearing. Briefly, the outer ear collects sounds and funnels them through the ear canal to the middle ear and eventually to the inner ear. The inner ear houses the cochlea, a snail-like organ that contains over 20,000 tiny hairs. Sound stimulates these hairs or hair cells and an electrical impulse is sent to the nerves that connect to the hair cells. The cochlea is set up in an organized fashion with the high pitches (frequencies) at one end and the low pitches at the other end. When sounds are made, only those hair cells that are "tuned" to those frequencies will set off the electrical impulse.

When a person is deaf, the number of hair cells is seriously reduced, so that an impulse cannot be sent. The cochlear implant attempts to replace this electrical activity in the cochlea by inserting electrodes to supply the missing electrical impulses to the nerves. Although the number of hair cells is very great, the number of electrodes placed in the cochlea can be as few as one or as many as twenty-four. These electrodes are tuned to different frequencies in a manner similar to the normal ear, i.e., the high pitches at one end and the low pitches at the other end. When a sound is made only those electrodes that are tuned to those frequencies will be activated. The signal then takes the traditional path to the brain. At the current time, there are three different multichannel cochlear implants available in the United States. More discussion of the different types of implants is provided in chapter 3.

What type of evaluation is needed to determine if the child is a candidate?

A child will require a battery of tests in order to determine whether he or she is a good candidate for a cochlear implant. Parents must realize that the cochlear implant evaluation, as a rule, extends through a period that ranges from several weeks to months. Comprehensive candidacy evaluation often requires multiple visits to the center, especially if the child is very young. A medical evaluation, CT scans of the ears, specialized audiological tests, and a speech/language assessment will be performed. Some centers conduct an educational evaluation, and some also perform an ophthalmologic, neurological, or psychological assessment, depending on the child's needs. Once all team members have evaluated the child, they meet to discuss their findings. The team makes a decision regarding implant candidacy and communicates it to the parents. A detailed description of a pre-implant evaluation appears in the following chapter.

What should I know about surgery and hospitalization?

The surgeon will carefully review the benefits and risks of implant surgery with parents at the time of the medical/surgical evaluation. Often, however, another team member will provide additional information about the general procedures related to surgery. This includes information about the length of stay in the hospital, the overnight care arrangements, the immediate pre- and postoperative requirements, and the individual policies of the hospital. (Chapter 4 is devoted to surgery and related issues.) In general, parents find this period extremely stressful, so they should inquire about the degree of support available during this time.

What does a child hear with an implant?

Although no one really knows what implant users hear, implants provide more sound for profoundly deaf individuals than traditional hearing aids do. Implants can deliver high-frequency sounds that were never available with conventional amplification. What any individual user does with this sound is variable. Children learn to use sound delivered by a cochlear implant over time with different degrees of success.

What are the educational/therapeutic needs of children with implants?

Children with implants come from a variety of educational and communication backgrounds. Some implant teams require a specific type of therapy after implantation. Some facilities do not accept children unless the parents make a full-time commitment to oral education. Others embrace a variety of educational and communication settings. During the discussion regarding educational support, parents should determine if anyone on the implant team serves as the educational liaison with their child's school. If so, that team member should meet the parents during the initial evaluation to plan communication with the school. Parents should also be aware of the level of post-implant educational support provided by the center.

In general, what are the long-term outcomes?

There is no guarantee that a particular level of benefit will occur after implantation. Parents should learn the general outcomes that have been observed in children with implants with respect to their auditory, speech, and educational achievements. When possible, more specific comparisons to children of similar age, duration of deafness, and other demographic factors can be presented. Parents must realize that **no definitive outcome can ever be promised**. A more comprehensive discussion of performance can be found in chapter 9.

What are the time and financial obligations of the parents?

Parents must learn the schedule of appointments that is required for both the pre-implant and post-implant stages. Families with two working parents should recognize that there is a substantial time commitment for follow-up, especially during the first year. Parents should obtain this schedule for device fittings and ongoing evaluations.

The family's financial obligations for the entire process should be discussed. Although most health insurers provide financial support for implantation, there is some variability across the country. Parents must investigate the reimbursement that their particular insurance carrier will provide and the restrictions the carrier may place on the implant center site, the surgeon, and/or the amount of follow-up services allowed. Each family should explore these restrictions early in the process to make certain there are no hidden, out-of-pocket expenses for which they are unprepared. All implant manufacturers have a reimbursement specialist to assist families with insurance issues.

How do the cochlear implant and Deaf culture coexist?

The implant center team should discuss with families issues of the Deaf community and its position with respect to cochlear implantation. Recently, the National Association for the Deaf (NAD), the largest organization that represents deaf individuals in the United States, reissued its position statement on implantation. While acknowledging that parents may choose implantation for their children, the NAD urges parents to value the Deaf community and what it represents. A copy of the NAD position statement can be found in Appendix B and further discussion of this topic can be found in chapter 10.

Although it is best to ascertain the answers to these questions before scheduling a candidacy evaluation, many parents begin the process with limited knowledge. Families may enter the pre-implant evaluation stage having already made the decision to implant and seek confirmation of the child's candidacy by the implant center team. Others may delay the final decision until more information is gathered. Regardless of how the family enters the pre-implant period, this time provides an opportunity for the implant center and the family to build and solidify a relationship.

Chapter 2

Candidacy Evaluation

Once a family enters the pre-implant period, they must then pass through a number of substages. The question of candidacy is crucial since it determines whether the child will continue through the process. A multidisciplinary team of professionals with expertise in the areas of audiology, speech, language, education, and medicine conducts the pre-implant evaluation. These professionals perform multiple tests within their individual disciplines to provide a comprehensive candidacy assessment. The sequence of appointments made for the pre-implant evaluation may vary from facility to facility as well as from patient to patient within a facility. In some cases, the parent may first meet with the cochlear implant surgeon who then refers the child for audiological testing. In other cases, the audiologist may be the point of entry into the implant protocol. Regardless of which professional is seen first, the child must meet certain audiological criteria in order to continue the process, thus making the audiologist the "gatekeeper" for candidacy. Once the audiological criteria have been met, teams perform additional evaluations to add to their pre-implant knowledge of the candidate.

Evaluating the Whole Child

One approach that has proved useful for many centers is a "whole child" orientation to implant candidacy. To assist in this undertaking, an evaluation tool known as the Children's Implant Profile, or ChIP, was developed in 1989 by the cochlear implant team at Manhattan Eye, Ear, and Throat Hospital. This profile assesses children across a variety of factors that have been shown to contribute to implant success. Each factor is rated along a continuum of concern ranging from "no concern" to "great concern." The ChIP provides the team and the family with a structured method of reviewing the components that may contribute to the child's performance with the device. The factors evaluated by the ChIP are explained in the following sections.

Age at Time of Implantation and Duration of Deafness

Two of the primary factors evaluated by the ChIP are age at time of implantation and duration of deafness. These are critically important because they identify the period of auditory deprivation and the point at which auditory stimulation begins. Children with short duration of profound deafness tend to perform better with cochlear implants than children with long duration of deafness. Thus congenitally deaf, or prelinguistically deafened children implanted at young ages, perform better than the same children implanted when they are older. Children born with mild or moderate hearing loss, progressing to profound hearing loss have been found to demonstrate good auditory skills with an implant. Hearing children who become profoundly deaf due to some cause like ototoxic drugs or head trauma will also perform well as long as they are implanted soon after losing their hearing.

In an effort to keep the duration of deafness as short as possible, more parents are seeking implantation for their infants as soon as the age criterion is met. In June 2000, the U.S. Food and Drug Administration (FDA) approved implantation in profoundly deaf children twelve months of age or older. Universal Newborn Hearing Screening has contributed to the phenomenon of infant implantation since identification can be made within days of an infant's birth. Many of the children identified at birth are then followed until they reach the criterion age. However, under cer-

---

Factors Evaluated on the Children's Implant Profile

☐ Age at Time of Implantation
☐ Duration of Deafness
☐ Medical/Radiological Assessment
☐ Handicapping Conditions
☐ Functional Hearing
☐ Speech and Language Abilities
☐ Family Structure and Support
☐ Level of Expectation
☐ Educational Environment and Availability of Support Services

---

tain medical circumstances, surgeons have the discretion to implant children *under* one year of age. This requires medical necessity and is not standard procedure at this time.

Medical/Radiological Assessment

Another category on the ChIP, medical/radiological assessment, is evaluated by the implant surgeon. Children must be able to undergo surgery and sustain at least two hours of general anesthesia. Therefore, surgery may have to be delayed in children with serious health issues until the other medical condition is resolved. For example, a child with a heart problem will not undergo implant surgery until his or her heart condition is addressed.

The radiological evaluation ensures that a cochlea is present. A small percentage of children are born without a cochlea, rendering them unable to benefit from cochlear implant technology. In other cases, the cochlea may be malformed or not fully developed. Malformations of the cochlea are often referred to as "Mondini deformities." These deformities can range in severity from a cochlea with fewer than the normal two-and-a-half turns to a condition known as a common cavity (in which the cochlea is present but there are no turns). Children with these types of malformations are capable of receiving a cochlear implant; performance outcomes for these and all children will be addressed in chapter 9.

Additional Disabilities

The presence of handicapping conditions may also affect the child's ability to use an implant to its fullest potential. Generally, children with noncognitive handicaps, such as blindness, can achieve good benefit from an implant (especially if the child is implanted at a young age and has a short duration of deafness). Children with handicaps that are cognitive in nature may show performance poorer than that of the average implant user. The level of cognitive handicap will influence the degree of benefit available to a particular child, thus, calling into question the wisdom of the decision to implant. Although children with autism, pervasive developmental delays (PDD), cerebral palsy, and even mild retardation have received implants, the range of performance for this group makes generalizations concerning outcomes almost impossible. Teams that implant children with cognitive or noncognitive handicaps often include professionals with expertise in these areas to advise them during the implant candidacy stage. These same professionals can provide valuable assistance during the period of post-implant habilitation.

Functional Hearing

As noted earlier, the audiologist often serves as the gatekeeper for entrance into the evaluation process. The child must undergo a comprehensive audiological evaluation in order to determine the effectiveness of the traditional amplification (hearing aid or FM) already in use. Trained pediatric audiologists use specially developed tests to measure the amount of speech a child is able to understand when listening only through a hearing aid or FM system. When young children have too little language to adequately assess their speech understanding, aided responses to pure tones are used as the criterion. If the auditory responses do not reach a certain level, the child is considered an implant candidate. When the child's performance with traditional amplification is similar to or better than that obtained by the average implant user, the child is not considered a candidate for implantation. All testing must be done using the best-fit hearing aids. If a child's hearing aids are inadequate, new ones will be recommended and a re-evaluation will take place after a period of use.

It should be noted that implant candidacy criteria have evolved substantially through the years as implant performance has improved. Children who were considered ineligible for implantation several years ago may now fit the new audiological standards that allow candidates to demonstrate some benefit from their conventional amplification. When implantation is not recommended due to the child's good functioning with hearing aids, it is suggested that parents return periodically to the implant center to determine if any change in audiological criteria has occurred. Advances in technology often result in a movement toward more relaxed audiological criteria, thus making a child eligible for an implant at a future time.

Speech and Language Abilities

A speech and language evaluation provides the implant team with valuable information about the child's current language competence, speech production, and overall communication ability as well as his or her potential for growth in these areas. Children should be assessed in their usual and customary mode of communication. For example, children who use sign language or Cued Speech for communication should be evaluated using that system.

21

Speech/language information obtained at the time of candidacy evaluation acts as a baseline from which the clinician can chart progress after implantation and make adjustments in therapy to accelerate that progress.

When the candidate is an infant, speech/language information is obtained using questionnaires that rely on parental reports. In addition, skilled professionals observe parent/child communication in naturalistic exchanges. Older children are evaluated using standardized materials. The goal of these evaluations is to identify the language age of the child, a measure of the formal language system in relationship to the child's chronological age.

Family Structure and Support

Implant facilities informally gauge family support, which is considered crucial to the child's success, by observing punctuality for appointments, the condition and wear time of hearing aids, and the interaction between parents and child. Reports of a child's attendance at early intervention sessions or school programs are also helpful.

Level of Expectation

Issues of family support are often linked to the level of expectation that parents and children have concerning implant performance. Implant centers determine parental expectations as part of the ChIP assessment; families with inappropriate expectations may view the implant as a cure-all that requires little or no effort beyond wearing the device. This sends a warning signal to the implant center team. In these cases, counseling for more appropriate device expectations is recommended. Adolescent candidates always require counseling in order to assess their level of expectation and to help them set appropriate goals.

Educational Environment and Availability of Support Services

It is important for local school professionals to be an integral part of the pre-implant process. The input of the child's teacher and speech/language therapist can assist the implant center in their educational assessment. Onsite visits by an educational consultant can ensure that helpful pre-implant information is gathered and proper post-implant therapy is available. Although a variety of educational environments can support children with implants, it is imperative for receiving schools to provide numerous listening and speaking opportunities throughout the school day. Children with cochlear implants who return to classrooms that do not challenge their listening and speaking abilities have only minimal success.

Making the Decision To Implant Your Child

The ChIP and other tools like it assist the implant center team in making a candidacy recommendation. This recommendation is then presented to the parents who make the final decision regarding implantation. Parents are advised to make this decision based on good quality information that reflects the individual needs of the child and the family lifestyle. Implantation must be approached with realistic goals by parents and children (when appropriate). Every child who receives a cochlear implant will not achieve the near-normal speech, language, and listening skills that many implant recipients enjoy. This reality must be factored into every parent's final decision.

The best outcome is reached when the team and the parents discuss each component of the evaluation and mutually agree upon the next step for the child. However, this does not always occur. In some circumstances, the implant team recommends implantation for the child but the parents do not

agree with the recommendation. Some parents defer the decision with the hope that technology will improve. In choosing to
wait, they preclude taking advantage of spoken language learning during the critical early years. That is their choice. In other
cases, the implant team may decide that the child would not make
an appropriate candidate due to the presence of confounding
problems. However, the family may disagree with this decision
and therefore, seek a second opinion. That, too, is their choice.
Responsible implant centers will respect the parents' decision
regardless of whether they agree or disagree with it. When parents and the implant center team are in agreement regarding the
appropriateness of an implant, the family can begin to explore
the differences between implant devices.

Chapter 3

Options in Implant Devices

Whether occurring simultaneously with the candidacy evaluation or after candidacy has been determined, a discussion of the types of implant devices available at the center is an important part of the pre-implant period. One of the choices to be considered during this time concerns the actual device that will be implanted. In some cases, the parent does not make the device selection because the cochlear implant center offers only one type of implant system. As noted in chapter 1, parents may wish to investigate the access a particular center has to the numerous types of technology before making a commitment to that center.

The number of cochlear implants on the market is far fewer than the number of hearing aids. Changes in hearing aid technology can be made more easily since there are no surgically implantable components. The fact that implantation involves surgery makes the choice a more critical one. Decisions regarding cochlear implant technology have more long-term ramifications since portions of the device are internally implanted. While there are more than forty manufacturers of hearing aids with hundreds of models to choose from, there are only three manufacturers of multichannel cochlear implant systems in the United States. Although each of these manufacturers would have you believe that its product is the best, the fact remains that no implant (or hearing aid) can guarantee a particular result. Fortunately, each cochlear implant system, regardless of manufacturer, provides children with adequate auditory information that can be processed meaningfully if properly fitted and supported.

Before describing each of the presently available cochlear implant systems, it is first important to review the basic components of cochlear implants. Every cochlear implant device is composed of internal and external parts. (See figure 3.1.)

The internal components are those that are surgically placed inside the head behind the ear. Electrodes, a receiver-stimulator (electronics that receive and deliver the signal), an antenna, and a magnet are all considered part of the internal workings of the device. These components can only be changed with additional surgery. The external portion of the implant consists of a microphone, speech processor, external transmitter and cord(s). Because these components are external, they can be easily replaced and upgraded as technology evolves.

Parents should keep in mind several issues when selecting a system for their child. Some of these may be more important for one family and their child than another. The internal components of the implant contain the electronics that interact with the external system. Therefore, selecting sophisticated internal technology is critically important since it cannot be readily changed. Consideration of the type of material that houses the receiver, MRI (Magnetic Resonance Imaging) compatibility, number of electrodes offered by the system, and overall reliability of the devices is also required. When considering external features, parents should investigate the size and outward appearance of the speech processor and headset, the software programs that are available to deliver speech to the internal receiver, the cost of maintaining the device over time, and the presence of accessories. The terms of the warranty and the level of company and/or center support for any given device require some assessment to assist parents in making the choice. Regardless, under no circumstances should a parent select a device for their child simply because the parent knows another child who has had success with the same type of implant. Nor should parents be swayed by either well-meaning professionals or other parents who have allegiance to

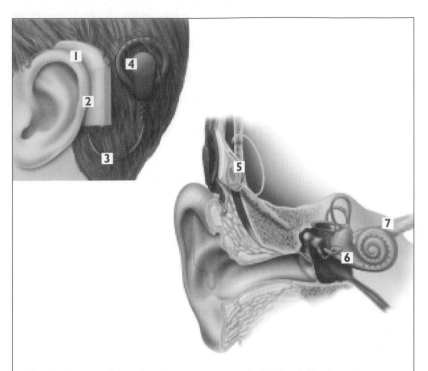

The Nucleus cochlear implant system works in the following manner:

1. Sounds are picked up by the small, directional microphone located in the ear level processor.

2. The speech processor filters, analyzes and digitizes the sound into coded signals.

3. The coded signals are sent from the speech processor to the transmitting coil.

4. The transmitting coil sends the coded signals as FM radio signals to the cochlear implant under the skin.

5. The cochlear implant delivers the appropriate electrical energy to the array of electrodes, which has been inserted into the cochlea.

6. The electrodes along the array stimulate the remaining auditory nerve fibers in the cochlea.

7. The resulting electrical sound information is sent through the auditory system to the brain for interpretation.

Pictures courtesy of Cochlear Ltd.

Figure 3.1. Internal and external components of a cochlear implant system and how it works.

a particular device. Device selection should be made based on an accumulation of information from a variety of sources.

Present-Day Devices

Although a single-channel implant (one that has only one electrode) is still manufactured in the United States under the name All Hear, it is not considered "state of the art" nor does it compete in performance with multichannel systems. Discussion will therefore be focused on only multichannel systems. The three manufacturers of multichannel cochlear implants in the United States are Cochlear Corporation, Advanced Bionics Corporation, and Med El Corporation. Each company has made a substantial commitment to the process of implantation through large capital investments in both research and design. Extensive information about the companies and their products can be obtained by visiting their websites or contacting their toll-free telephone numbers. A brief history of each company is provided here; the reader may wish to investigate further by accessing the resources in Appendix B.

Cochlear Corporation was the first company to manufacture and distribute multichannel cochlear implants in the world. For this reason, users of their device outnumber those of other manufacturers. The parent company is based in Australia, with the American headquarters located in Englewood, Colorado. The company has six subsidiaries around the world. Their products include the Nucleus 22 and the Nucleus 24 devices. The Nucleus 22 was the first multichannel cochlear implant system approved by the Food and Drug Administration (FDA) for use in the United States. This product was replaced by an updated version, known as the Nucleus 24 and, more recently, the Nucleus 24 RCS. The company supports more than 36,000 cochlear implant recipients speaking more than twenty-three different languages around the world.

Advanced Bionics Corporation, located in Sylmar, California, entered the cochlear implant field in 1995. At the time they appeared in the American marketplace, Cochlear Corporation was the sole manufacturer of multichannel implants. Advanced Bionics' presence in the industry substantially changed the face of implantation by adding a competitive force. This competition created an environment that enabled implant technology to grow exponentially in a very short period of time. Despite their short term in the industry, Advanced Bionics has developed markets in a number of different countries around the world. They support over 10,000 implants worldwide. Their product, known as the Clarion device, has been through several generations as new technological advances have been introduced. Their latest product is known as the C II.

Med El Corporation is based in Innsbruck, Austria, with its American subsidiary located in Raleigh, North Carolina. The leaders in Med El have been active in the field since the early 1980s when only single-channel devices were available. Their major market distribution was first in Europe. However, in 1994, they began distributing their device in the United States. Their product, known as the Med El device, has evolved from the early Combi 40 to the Tempo 40+. From fourteen international offices, they support 6,000 implant users in over 250 clinics in fifty-four countries worldwide.

All three cochlear implant systems have certain similarities and differences. Although each company will boast product superiority, no implant system restores hearing to normalcy and no system can unequivocally guarantee a particular result. There are many choices within and among the systems. Parents will be bombarded with information about different types of internal receivers, speech processing strategies, and accessories. In an effort to provide a text that will not become outdated as the technology changes, only a minimal description of each of the systems is presented here. The intent is to provide parents with questions (and reasons for these questions) so a meaningful discussion of devices can occur.

Internal Components

The *internal receiver* of cochlear implant systems can be made from a variety of materials. The first question a parent should ask concerns the types of materials that make up an individual system. The Nucleus system is encased in *silicone* while the Clarion and Med El systems are encased in *ceramic*. There are certain advantages and disadvantages to each. Those that are encased in silicone are more flexible, conform to the skull more easily, and are generally thinner than those that are encased in ceramic. A parent might then ask, "Why ceramic?" Ceramic casings protect the internal components, (especially the antenna) from damage and transmit the signal more efficiently. However, the ceramic casings tend to be somewhat thicker and less flexible. Because of their thickness, more drilling is required during surgery so that the implant has a flatter profile on the skull. Both silicone- and ceramic-encased internal receivers work well; both have their inherent problems. Any direct blow to the head in the area of the implant can result in damage to the internal receiver, regardless of whether it is silicone or ceramic. If this occurs, the child must undergo another surgery to replace the damaged implant.

Electrodes are also part of the internal components of the system. The electrodes are important because they actively deliver the signal to the cochlear nerve endings. There is no magic number of electrodes that an implant must have (although more than one is needed for good speech understanding to occur). Parents often think that the more electrodes there are, the better

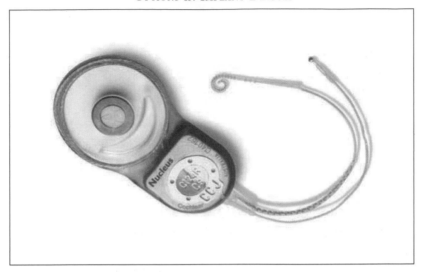

Figure 3.2. The Nucleus 24 internal electrode array

the device. The number of electrodes within the present-day systems is actually quite similar, ranging from sixteen to twenty-four. Each of the systems delivers information to these electrodes in a specific way. The manner in which the electrodes fire contributes to the different individual speech processing strategies. (More information on speech processing strategies can be found later in this chapter.)

The electrode can also differ in the *shape of its array*. Some electrode arrays are *straight* (e.g., Med El) while others are *precoiled* (e.g., Clarion and Nucleus 24 RCS). (See figures 3.2, 3.3, and 3.4.) Precoiled arrays were developed to follow the natural snail-like shape of the cochlea. The implant designers believed that this type of stimulation reduces the power needed to run the implant and brings the electrode closer to nerve endings. This configuration may result in better performance; however, since all three implants report excellent results, the precoiled shape may not be as critical as believed. Future electrode designs may make array shape more important.

Parents must also consider other characteristics of the internal components of cochlear implants. These include the *MRI*

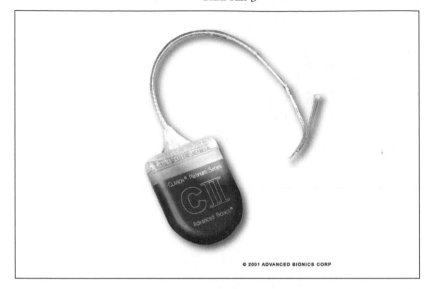

© 2001 ADVANCED BIONICS CORP

Figure 3.3. The Advanced Bionics CII internal electrode array

compatibility of the device and the presence of certain electronic features known as *telemetry*. An MRI is a type of X-ray technology that uses magnets to take pictures inside the body, usually to detect tumors or assess damage to tissue. Since the MRI uses magnets, and the implant has a magnet and other types of materials that are attracted by magnets, the MRI is not generally recommended for individuals with implants. Some devices are considered MRI-compatible (Nucleus 24 and 24 RCS) while others (Clarion, Med El, Nucleus 22) require certain precautions if an MRI is necessary. Parents might ask, "How can a device with a magnet inside be considered MRI-compatible?" This is accomplished in two ways. First, the internal components can be composed of a material that is not attracted by magnets (these are known as nonferrous materials). Second, the actual magnet inside can be removed if an MRI is required. Removal of the magnet involves injecting the area with a local anesthetic, making an incision, and temporarily removing the magnet. Once the MRI is completed, the magnet is replaced and the area is closed with stitches.

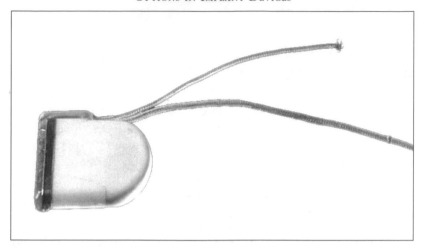

Figure 3.4. Med El internal electrode array

What happens when a child has a device that is not MRI-compatible? A child can undergo an MRI with certain restrictions. First, the type of MRI machine must be one that delivers 1.5 teslas or less of power. (Teslas are a measure of the strength of the magnet in an MRI system.) Second, the area of the implant should be bandaged tightly so the magnetic pull does not move the internal device too much. Fortunately, in most cases, other types of X-rays can be used thereby forgoing the MRI altogether and decreasing the incidence of any problem.

Availability of a *telemetry* system in the internal components of an implant is important. Telemetry is a remote method of measuring the electrical response of the device. In other words, it permits the audiologist to make certain decisions about how well the internal receiver is working. There are two types of telemetry systems. One is known as *impedance telemetry*. This type of telemetry checks the internal receiver to determine if the electrodes are functioning according to specification. Why is this type of telemetry necessary? Impedance telemetry permits the audiologist to monitor the internal device each time the child comes to the center after implantation. All of the newer systems have this type of telemetry.

Neural Response Telemetry (NRT) is a type of telemetry that measures the response of the auditory nerve at each electrode placement. NRT can be used to assist in setting the device with very young children. The Nucleus 24 currently has this type of telemetry. The Clarion C II will also incorporate a similar system in its future device. The uses of NRT are just beginning to be explored and may provide additional information about electrodes and the nerve populations they stimulate.

Before leaving the discussion of the internal receiver, it should be noted that the internal and external components must work together to provide the best signal to the cochlea. *Speech processing strategies* are the link between the external and internal portions of the implant system. They are the "directions" that provide the internal receiver with information about the sounds that are occurring. There are different types of speech processing strategies. During the device counseling session, parents should ask, "What speech processing strategies does the implant provide?" The following description is fundamental and may not answer questions for parents who are interested in more detail. For an in-depth discussion about speech processing strategies, parents may wish to read further. (See references in Appendix B.)

A basic principle of speech processing is that no strategy delivers the same amount of benefit to every implant user. Thus, there are a variety of strategies available within and among the implant systems. These function by delivering information to the electrodes based on a formula designed specifically for each device. Speech processing strategies include: CIS (Continuous Interleaved Sampling), SPEAK (Spectral Peak), ACE (Advanced Combined Encoder), SAS (Simultaneous Analog Stimulation), PPS (Paired Pulsatile Stimulation), and N of M (N meaning the number of electrodes stimulated across M channels). CIS is available on the Clarion, Nucleus 24, and Med El devices. However, the CIS of Clarion is not exactly the same as the CIS of Nucleus or the CIS of Med El. SPEAK and ACE are available on the Nucleus 24 system. SAS and PPS are available on the Clarion, and N of M is accessible through the Med El. It is crucial that a variety of strategies be available on any one device so that a child can have access to the strategy that will work best for him or her. Parents should discuss each of these strategies with their implant center audiologist.

External Components

The external components of the cochlear implant system include the speech processor and the features that are incorporated in it and the microphone/headset. The speech processor is that portion of the system that houses the electronics of the external unit. It can be either body-worn (typically the size of a pager) or worn behind the ear, similar to a conventional behind-the-ear (BTE) hearing aid. Each of the manufacturers offers both a body and BTE configuration. There are certain advantages and disadvantages to each. Clearly, body-worn devices are bulkier and less cosmetically appealing (especially for teenagers). However, they are more efficient to operate, they are less likely to be damaged or lost, and they often have more capabilities than the smaller BTE versions.

Body-worn units are more efficient to operate because the power supply is often a rechargeable AA battery (Nucleus and Med El) or a special rechargeable battery manufactured by the company (Clarion). These batteries often last 15 hours, and they are simple and inexpensive to recharge. Body-worn units are less subject to damage or loss because of their overall size and the manner in which they are worn. The majority of young children uses body processors and wear them on their back under clothing in specially designed harnesses. This prevents the device from

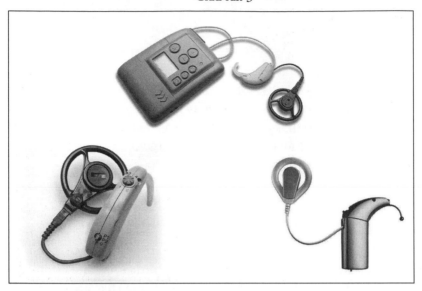

Figure 3.5. Nucleus 24 speech processors

being damaged by everyday mishaps such as spilled water or juice. Since the device is worn under the clothing, it is virtually impossible for it to fall off and become lost.

Another feature that will vary somewhat among body-worn processors is the microphone headset. This portion of the device consists of the microphone and external transmitter. It is located on the head and makes contact with the internal receiver through magnetic attraction. Some manufacturers (Med El, Nucleus) have a headset that consists of two pieces—a portion that sits behind the ear and houses the microphone and a portion that contains the transmitter and magnet to hold it on the head. Clarion body processors have a slightly different headset arrangement. The microphone, transmitter, and magnet are contained in a single unit. In other words, there is no portion that sits behind the ear. (See figures 3.5, 3.6, and 3.7.)

The physical size of the body processor allows it to house more features. These features might include more memory, more variety of speech processing strategies, or more accessories. Parents

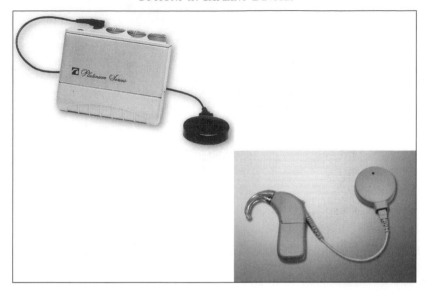

Figure 3.6. Advanced Bionics speech processors

might then question, "Why would I use a BTE model with my child?" The most obvious appeal for choosing the BTE processor has to do with overall size. For adolescents who are concerned about appearances, an implant may be unacceptable unless it is a BTE model. With very active young children, however, these smaller units can easily dislodge and be lost. The expense of replacing a lost external device can become costly. Additionally, in some BTE processors (Nucleus, Med El), power is supplied through traditional button-type hearing aid batteries. These are not rechargeable and may have to be changed more often, thus introducing battery cost as a possible concern. One BTE processor (Clarion) uses a specially designed rechargeable battery. However, it too must be replaced with another rechargeable battery after several hours of use.

Given all the available options, parents may wonder, "Do I have to decide which size device I want for my child at the time of his or her surgery?" In most cases, parents need not worry. The majority of cochlear implant facilities purchase the implants

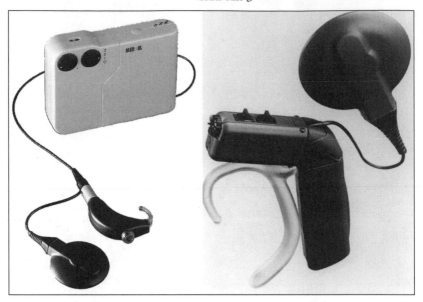

Figure 3.7. Med El speech processors

as a package; that is, the child receives both the body-worn and the BTE unit. However, some centers do not provide both a body and a BTE external system. It is important to ask about this issue when choosing a particular center.

Parents should explore features other than size that are offered by each implant system. Body and BTE processors can only store a certain amount of information in their memories. These memory stores are known as the program selectors. Parents might ask, "What does a program selector do and why is it important?" A program selector can be thought of as a filing cabinet in which specific information about a particular speech processing strategy can be placed. This information is what makes up the child's MAP. (A further discussion of mapping is included in chapter 5.) The MAP directs the speech processing strategy so that it delivers sound at a comfortable level for the child. Program selectors allow the audiologist to place more than one MAP in the speech processor. All present-day devices are capable of multiple MAP storage. Body-worn processors can hold either three or four programs; BTE processors can hold either two or three programs.

In addition to multiple MAP storage, each device provides a method of adjusting the sensitivity and the volume of the implant system. Controls help the implant user to make sounds louder or softer (volume control) and decrease or increase the amount of sound the microphone can detect (sensitivity control). Devices have minor differences in the location and type of these controls. Body processors have easy-to-operate dials or buttons that can be set so that young children cannot play with them. Smaller BTE models may not have the same number and type of controls as the larger body-worn units.

Accessories and Features

Each of the cochlear implant systems provides accessories that may be attractive to individual users. *Microphone-monitoring* systems that are built into the processor are available with some body-worn units (Nucleus, Clarion). This feature allows parents to use specially designed headphones to listen to the child's microphone to determine if it is functioning properly. In addition, audible alarms that signal that a battery is losing power can be activated on some body units (Clarion, Nucleus). As a further option, the Nucleus body unit offers a personal alarm system that is audible only to the user. In the Clarion devices, an easily heard signal alerts parents when the external headset has fallen from the child's head.

All devices, both body and BTE, are compatible with a variety of FM units. Special adapter cords are required to interface the two systems. It is important that parents discuss the connection of implants and FM systems with the professionals at their implant facility and educational setting.

Warranties and Maintenance

Each company guarantees the internal receiver for a period of ten years and the external speech processor for three years. Once the warranty period for the external equipment expires, the companies offer a service contract to cover any future repairs. Cochlear Corporation offers a unique warranty that replaces one speech processor free of charge if it is lost or stolen during the warranty period. Otherwise, parents can purchase a separate contract from outside sources for this purpose.

Maintenance of the cochlear implant system is minimal over time. Batteries and cords are not covered under warranty and must be replaced periodically at the family's expense. The cost of replacing these items is reasonable. Proper upkeep of the external equipment will ensure its functioning over time. Implant center personnel will discuss routine maintenance procedures to keep the device in optimal working condition.

In choosing a particular device, healthy skepticism should be maintained when recommendations come directly from manufacturers, since their goal is to market a product. Parents should contact the manufacturers, but information gleaned from them should be discussed with a variety of professionals to separate "hype" from fact. Other parents whose children have already received implants can be an additional resource. They may be able to inform new parents about some of the strengths and weaknesses of their own child's device.

The good news for parents is that if a child is an appropriate implant candidate, any of the devices will provide information to assist in the development of listening skills. In the final analysis, it is important for parents to understand the differences among devices and be comfortable with the device choice they ultimately make.

Chapter 4

The Surgical Stage

Once the decision to implant has been made and the device selected, the parents and child enter the next stage, the surgical stage. This period often creates the most stress for parents since *all* surgery carries with it certain risks. Parents meet with the surgeon to discuss these surgical risks and ask questions that may have arisen during the evaluation period. When meeting with parents, surgeons often begin with a review of the anatomy and physiology of the ear and how the implant works. The type of surgery performed for a cochlear implant is known as a tympanomastoidectomy. This surgical procedure has been in existence for many years and was used extensively for medical intervention before the development of the implant. There are many articles that are published in medical journals that describe this surgery in detail. A brief description of the surgical process follows to provide parents with background knowledge from which they can make additional queries. The general surgical procedure in use today is globally accepted, although there are slight variations both within the United States and around the world.

The Surgical Process

During the evaluation stage, parents should receive a thorough presentation on the implant surgery and what it entails, including
- presurgical blood work-up and medical evaluation,
- hospital policies concerning pediatric patients,
- implant facility recommendations,

- types and risks of anesthesia,
- other risks associated with surgery,
- general timeline of events,
- description of the surgery,
- preparing the child for the surgical experience,
- immediate postoperative sequelae (consequences), and
- postsurgical care.

Presurgical Blood Work-Up and Medical Evaluation

Parents are advised to take their child to the pediatrician to ensure the child's general health and well-being in advance of surgery. Blood tests are required before surgery to rule out any serious infections. Although individual physicians may have different requirements, blood is usually drawn a week prior to surgery. Results of these blood tests must be available on the day of surgery. The surgeon must be alerted if the child is taking medications at the time of surgery.

Hospital Policies Concerning Pediatric Patients

Each hospital has certain rules regarding the presence of parents in the holding area (area just outside the operating room), the operating room, and on the ward. Parents should understand these rules before the child is hospitalized. Often, facilities have videos that children can view that may use cartoonlike characters or puppets to explain the procedures and describe the surroundings. Arrangements for special dietary needs, assistive devices, or interpreters should be made before admission to ensure their availability.

Implant Facility Recommendations

Many implant facilities will make general recommendations they have found invaluable through experiences with other patients. For example, since the child often leaves the hospital with a pressure bandage over the operated ear, parents should bring a button-down shirt instead of a pullover shirt for the child to wear home. For children who wear glasses, removing the temple bar from an old pair can make it easier for the child after surgery. Obviously, bringing a child's favorite stuffed animal, doll, or blanket is always recommended. Sometimes an implant team member will bandage the doll or stuffed animal's ear with the same large bandage, so the child has a partner who has shared in the procedure. Some implant manufacturers provide a stuffed animal for the child to receive after surgery.

Types and Risks of Anesthesia

Any surgery carries with it certain risks related to anesthesia. Cochlear implant surgery is performed under general anesthesia. This requires that the child be placed in a deep sleep state. Prior to the surgery, parents will have the opportunity to meet with the anesthesiologist, (when possible, a pediatric anesthesiologist) to report any allergies or medical issues that are pertinent to the child. The anesthesiologist will also answer any questions parents have concerning the type of anesthesia and the most common after-effects. It is often helpful for parents to discuss their fears about anesthesia with parents of children who have already been through the procedure. This is a time during which the support of other parents can be most helpful.

Other Risks Associated with Surgery

In addition to anesthesia issues, certain risks are inherent in cochlear implant surgery. Since the surgical site is close to the facial nerve, there is always a very small risk that the nerve may be damaged. A facial nerve monitor keeps track of the status of the nerve during surgery. The incidence of facial nerve damage has been infrequent, but families considering surgery need to be informed of its possibility. In some cases, the child may experience mild facial nerve weakness after surgery. This is usually temporary with no apparent long-term effect. Other risks include postoperative infection and dizziness, which, if they occur, resolve rapidly over time. In very rare cases, there is the possibility of postoperative meningitis. The incidence of this occurrence has been negligible.

General Timeline of Events

Parents should be aware of the general sequence of surgical events and the duration of the surgery itself. In the United States, children are admitted to the hospital on the morning of the procedure. In most cases, the surgery will last approximately two to four hours. Once the surgery is completed, the child will stay in the recovery room for another one to two hours, depending on the time spent under general anesthesia. Once out of the recovery room, the child is transported back to a room on the ward. In most cases, the child remains in the hospital overnight and is discharged the next morning. In many cases, the child returns to the surgeon's office within a week after the surgery for a post-surgical visit so that the healing of the implant site can be assessed. If an appointment for the initial switch-on has not already been made, it is likely to be scheduled at this time.

Description of the Surgery

The preparation for surgery begins with dressing the child in the surgical gown. For some toddlers who are resistant to changing clothes, this can create unnecessary tension early on in the process. If dressing issues are known to provoke negative behaviors, parents may wish to desensitize the child in advance of the surgery by making it a game or providing a tangible reward. If this cannot be accomplished, then parents should be prepared for the battle so that it does not add to their stress level on that day.

After the child is appropriately gowned, he or she is transported to the operating room. (In some cases, pre-sedation may be administered in the room prior to departure for the surgical suite.) Upon arrival on the surgical floor, the child may be situated in a holding area or small room outside the operating theatre to await surgery. Some hospitals allow parents to remain with the child in this area. Some may also permit one parent to enter the surgical suite and remain with the child until sedated. Policies vary from hospital to hospital, and it is best to discuss these matters with the implant team in advance to learn hospital policy. Parents are not permitted to remain in the surgical suite during the procedure.

During the surgical procedure, parents often stay in a surgical waiting area. Most doctors recommend that parents remain close to the designated area in the unlikely event that the surgeon requires a consultation during the procedure. These may be the most stressful hours that parents will spend during the entire implant process. It is sometimes helpful when a patient liaison or another parent can lend support through this period. If possible, even the occasional presence of a team member during this time can help relieve parental tension.

Once inside the operating suite, the child receives general anesthesia and the head is prepared for the surgery. The area around the ear is usually shaved. (Note that some surgeons no longer shave the head.) An incision is made behind the ear in order to access the site where the implant will be inserted. The size and shape of the incision will vary with the surgeon's preference. (When meeting with the surgeon prior to implant surgery, parents may wish to inquire about the type of incision that will be made.) The surgeon then drills into the mastoid (behind the ear) to enter the area known as the facial recess. This allows access to the cochlea. Once the surgeon has identified the cochlea, he or she will insert the electrodes and secure the receiver-stimulator portion of the device. Before closing the incision, the device will be tested through the telemetry system to ensure that it is functioning properly. A large pressure bandage is then placed over the ear, and the child is then moved to the recovery room.

Some hospitals allow parents to be with the child in the recovery room after surgery. Other hospitals do not permit parents in this area. Again, it is best to check with the implant facility to determine the exact policy. Once out of recovery, the child is brought back to the room on the hospital ward.

Preparing the Child for the Surgical Experience

As soon as parents have an understanding of the surgical process, it is important to convey this information to the child. A description of surgery should be presented at an appropriate linguistic level for the child. Obviously, for older children, a frank discussion of the sequence of pre- and postsurgical events is possible. For younger children, booklets distributed by the device manufacturers are available to assist in this counseling. Some implant teams use dolls or stuffed animals to play-act the surgical events for the young child. It is extremely important that all children (except for infants) be exposed to some facts about the procedure. This information can be reinforced with assistance from the school program, the therapists working with the child, and the parents.

Immediate Postoperative Sequelae (Consequences)

Most children will sleep for several hours after surgery. They may awaken and be uncomfortable initially. They may whine, cry, and/or be very clingy. A small percentage of children may vomit after surgery. This is usually a result of general anesthesia and passes quickly. Some of the older children report being dizzy or light-headed. This sensation also tends to pass with time. The majority of children awaken after several hours without any symptoms. In fact, parents often remark about the child's resiliency after undergoing the procedure.

Postsurgical Care

Although individual differences exist among surgeons, there are some general guidelines for postoperative care following implantation. The large bandage can usually be removed within twenty-four to forty-eight hours after discharge from the hospital. Parents are advised not to get the surgical site wet for a specified period of time. This restriction will vary from surgeon to surgeon and may be as short as two days or as long as a week. Children must continue taking the antibiotics that were prescribed as a precautionary measure during the hospitalization until all medication is consumed. On the rare occasions when children have discomfort, over-the-counter pain relievers are recommended. The child can resume normal activity once he or she returns home; however, it is preferred that playground supervision be provided at school. Some implant teams may place other restrictions on the child. Usually, the teams and surgeons provide these postoperative instructions to parents in written form for future reference.

Waiting for Device Activation

The normal course of recovery for children after implantation is usually uneventful. However, parents are instructed to contact the surgeon or implant center if any questions or concerns should arise. Following clearance from the surgeon, the family is scheduled to return to the implant facility approximately one month after the surgery to begin the next phase of the process, the post-implantation stage.

Although the stress of the actual surgery has ended at this juncture, parents may find it helpful to have ongoing contact with the implant center team or another parent. The month-long period of waiting for the initial device switch-on is often filled with new tensions about the success of implant surgery. The school can also assist the implant center in providing support for the parents during this interval. It is important that parents do not feel abandoned during this downtime that occurs between surgery and activation.

Many centers provide parents with the external components of the implant system and encourage them to read the manufacturers' booklets about the equipment and accessories before they arrive for device activation. This provides parents with information about the various parts of the implant so that they can become familiar with the terms that will be used on the day of switch-on. This knowledge empowers parents to be active participants rather than passive observers on the day of device activation.

Chapter 5

The Post-Implantation Stage:
Initial Switch-On and Counseling about Device Maintenance

Parents and children often approach the period known as the initial switch-on or tune-up with a great deal of anticipation and anxiety. The waiting period of approximately one month after surgery is often filled with feelings that range from excitement to doubt. For this reason, it is important for parents and child to have a complete understanding of the initial switch-on experience so that the range of responses that are possible is clearly understood. It is much more productive for the audiologist working with the child to explain everything that will happen before beginning the process rather than explaining it as it occurs.

The switch-on, or initial tune-up, usually takes place over a two-day period during which the device is activated and the parents learn how to manage the equipment. Individual centers have developed their own calendars for switch-on, so the time span and sequence of activities may differ from center to center. Regardless of the exact schedule, a number of tasks have to be done during this initial period of activation, including:

- dispensing and fitting the child with the external equipment and accessories,
- adjusting the electrical levels,
- assessing the initial auditory responses with the implant, and
- counseling parents, implant recipients, and caregivers about the maintenance of the system.

Initial Switch-On

Dispensing and Fitting the Child
with the External Equipment and Accessories

When the switch-on begins, the child is wearing the external equipment that is attached via a cable to the programming station and computer. (See figure 5.1.) This effectively connects the implanted portion of the device with the external portion of the system. Young implant recipients require two audiologists working together during the session. A programming audiologist sits at the computer and makes adjustments to the device through special computer software. The other audiologist works directly with the child to monitor auditory responsiveness. This test environment is not unlike a traditional audiological assessment in which one audiologist sits at the audiometer and the other sits with the child to assist with the listening task. However, unlike an audiological evaluation, the programming session does not have to be done in a soundproof room. For young children especially, it is important that they be in a friendly, non-threatening environment. For this reason, it is not unusual to see numerous toys, games, and videos in switch-on rooms.

In order to link the total implant system to the computer, the child must wear the headset. This portion consists of the microphone, magnet, and transmitter. When the external magnet on the transmitter is placed near the implanted magnet of the receiver, the two components will connect easily. This allows the audiologist access to the electrodes implanted in the cochlea. Under most circumstances, getting the child to wear the headset for the first time takes only a few seconds. However, toddlers sometimes show initial resistance. This should come as no surprise to anyone who has ever parented a two-year-old. Often

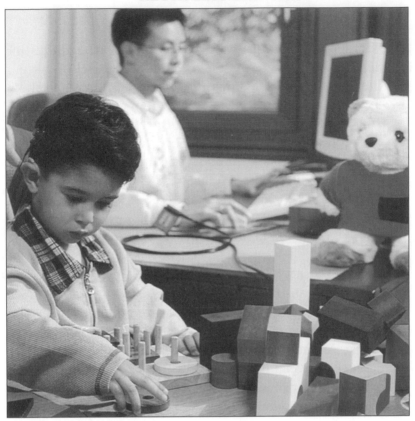

Figure 5.1. Child connected to programming station and equipment

distraction techniques, which engage the child in some other activity, enable the audiologist to put the headset in place. Experience suggests that even the most reluctant child will eventually wear the external equipment after a brief period of acclimation.

Adjusting the Electrical Levels

Once all the external and internal components are linked, the process of setting the electrodes begins. The programming audiologist activates each of the individual implanted electrodes one at a time. The purpose of this procedure is to determine the level of electrical stimulation that each electrode requires for producing a response in the child. The lowest level of current that is needed to get an auditory response is called the threshold or *T-level*. These responses can be conditioned responses (e.g., the child responds to the stimulated electrode by placing a block in a bucket or a peg in a board) or observed responses (such as eye movement). Implant devices, which incorporate a system known as Neural Response Telemetry (NRT) (described in chapter 3), enable the clinician to obtain these measures in a more objective manner. NRT has proven to be a reliable tool for programming implants in children too young to provide feedback during tuning.

After all T-levels have been obtained, the programmer then works on setting the comfort level or *C-level*. (This is sometimes referred to as the M-level, as in the most comfortable level.) The C-level represents the level of current that creates a sensation of sound that is comfortably loud. This is an important value since the distance between the T-level and C-level for each electrode will provide the dynamic range of the implant. The dynamic range is the amount that sound is allowed to grow from its softest to its loudest. A good dynamic range is one that permits sound to grow evenly from soft to loud. If the dynamic range is very narrow, sound does not grow in the appropriate manner. This restricts auditory perception. It is not unusual, however, for children to show narrow ranges at the time of the initial switch-on. Parents can be assured that this range will grow with time as the child adapts to the implant and the sound it delivers.

When each electrode has been assessed for a T- and a C-level, the computer then generates a MAP. The MAP records the information detailing the current levels for each electrode. It is unique to each child with a cochlear implant. No child should ever use another child's processor because the MAPs within it are different. MAPs are stored on a computer chip located in the speech processor using a retrieval system similar to a file cabinet. Each drawer in the file cabinet is called a program. One MAP is assigned to a single program. Over time, the audiologist will create new MAPs, erase old MAPs from the program slot, and replace them with the newer versions. All current implants are able to store more than one MAP on the speech processor. Return trips to the implant center may be less frequent because of this feature. Access to multiple MAPs enables the parent to make comparisons between and among the different programs that are stored in the speech processor.

Once all T- and C-levels have been found and a MAP has been generated, the child is finally given an opportunity to listen to speech. This is the moment that parents have anticipated and played out in their minds. It is difficult to predict what any given child's first response to speech through the implant will be. A child's reaction is related to his or her age and prior experience with listening through hearing aids. It is not unusual for some children to show very little response, especially if they are very young. In some cases, the child's first response to sound may disappoint the parents. Some children may cry or attempt to remove the headset. Parents should know that any crying is more likely to be a reaction to an unfamiliar stimulus and not to pain. Nonetheless, parents will often find the experience unsettling and may begin to second-guess their decision about implantation. Parents should trust the judgments of the implant center team; the team has experience with the range of responses seen at initial switch-on and should continue their work even if a negative response occurs.

Assessing the Initial Auditory Responses with the Implant

Most children show observable responses to speech during the switch-on session. Parents should understand that these responses do not generalize to everyday activities until wear time and training has occurred. The audiologist may perform some simple post-switch-on listening assessments to determine which auditory skills are present. The audiologist can then identify those skills that should be targeted by the school program or therapist working with the child. Parents are encouraged to view the initial switch-on as the starting point in the child's auditory development. It is a beginning, not an end.

Counseling Parents, Implant Recipients, and Caregivers about the Maintenance of the System

Before leaving the implant facility on the day of the initial switch-on, parents receive directions on how the device works and how to check that it is functioning properly. These discussions might also include teachers, therapists, caregivers, grandparents, siblings, and the implant recipient. Whoever is in direct contact with the child should have some knowledge of the care and management of the implant. It follows then, that individuals who have regular contact with the implant recipient must have in-depth knowledge of how the device functions. The following issues are generally reviewed during this session:
- wearing the cochlear implant,
- turning the device on and off,
- setting the volume and sensitivity controls,
- mapping beyond the initial switch-on,
- changing programs,
- battery maintenance,
- checking microphone function,
- checking the cords,
- performing daily listening and visual checks of the system,
- alarms, lights, and icons,
- precautions regarding static electricity,
- precautions regarding moisture,
- MRI issues,
- cordless telephones, airports, and security systems,

- physical activity,
- medical precautions, and
- contacting the implant center for replacement equipment or other emergencies.

Wearing the Cochlear Implant

Very young children cannot be expected to protect their body-worn processor, so they wear a harness that holds it either on their back or on their chest. Back placement is recommended so that the device is out of the child's reach and is also protected from exposure to the everyday bumps and grinds of toddler life. They should not wear the device attached to their pants belt. This arrangement can be problematic when the belt is loosened for trips to the bathroom. Wearing the device on the belt exposes the processor to more damaging possibilities. Older children often wear their processors in small packs around their waist; manufacturers provide these as part of the accessory package. For some vigorous sports, such as football, hockey, or rugby, older children may want to remove their body-worn processors as well as their headsets as a precaution against damage. The external parts of the system should also be removed for water sports such as swimming and snorkeling.

The availability of behind-the-ear (BTE) speech processors creates new challenges in wearing the device. Most very young children do not use ear-level processors. However, there may be certain occasions for which parents choose this less conspicuous device. For those circumstances, it is important that the case of the speech processor be secured to the ear by an earmold, huggie, or, in some cases, a tether that attaches to the clothing. This guards against loss of the device for the active toddler who may be wearing it.

Turning the Device On and Off

Each implant has an on/off dial or button. Parents are instructed in the proper sequence of turning the device on each morning. They can adjust the volume and sensitivity controls (see below) to ensure that their child begins the day with the device comfortably set. Some implants have the capacity to lock out all the controls, thereby preventing young children from manipulating them or turning the device off.

Setting the Volume and Sensitivity Controls

Through a series of external controls, the child, parent, teacher, or therapist can adjust the volume and sensitivity of the unit. Most parents are familiar with volume controls from the use of the child's FM or hearing aid. These act in a similar manner on the cochlear implant. The volume control increases or decreases the loudness of the signal coming into the speech processor. Most parents, however, are not familiar with the concept of sensitivity adjustment. The sensitivity regulator changes the microphone's ability to detect sounds that are either far away or close by. Think of the sensitivity control as a "bubble" around the implant user. If the sensitivity is set at a low level, the bubble is small and the microphone works best at detecting those signals inside the bubble. If the sensitivity is set at a high level, the bubble is larger and the microphone accesses sounds from a greater distance. Sounds outside the bubble may still be heard, but they will be softer in relation to the sounds inside the bubble. Each type of implant sets sensitivity by using units specific to that device. An implant center staff member will explain how to adjust the sensitivity of any given implant system and recommend appropriate settings for everyday use. It is important for parents, teachers, therapists, and, when appropriate, implant users to know about these settings to ensure that the device delivers the maximum amount of sound for a given situation.

Mapping Beyond the Initial Switch-On

MAPs will need to be changed periodically for as long as the child wears the implant. MAP adjustments occur more frequently during the first year of implantation than in subsequent years. Too many or too few MAP changes are not productive. When MAPs are changed too frequently, the child may not have enough time to adapt to sound. When MAPs are changed too infrequently, the child may be using a MAP that is not delivering enough sound to his or her auditory system. Parents are sometimes fearful that they will not recognize when a MAP change is required. More often than not, parents become expert in determining the need for a new MAP, since their daily interactions provide them with a baseline of performance from which to make this judgment. For example, parents may notice that their child is no longer responding to his or her name consistently. Parents who are unsure of their child's mapping needs may contact the implant facility to help determine if the child will benefit from a new MAP.

Children return to the cochlear implant center then, on a regular basis, for re-mappings of the speech processor. The schedule of these appointments varies and is set by the individual implant facility. Generally, younger children return monthly during the first year of implant use; older children may require less-frequent re-mapping. At each mapping session after the initial switch-on, the child will receive two, three, or four MAPs (depending upon the type of device) to use over a period of time.

Changing Programs

Because the new generation of implant devices allows different MAPs to be placed in the assorted program slots in the speech processor, parents can change programs at home without returning to the implant center. During the interval between mapping sessions at the center, parents are responsible for monitoring the child's performance over time with each of the programs. Changing from one program to the next often requires just pressing a button, turning a control dial, or moving a toggle switch. When parents switch from one MAP to the next, several performance outcomes are possible. There may be no change, a positive change, or a negative change in the auditory or speech skills of the child. If parents do not observe immediate changes, they should continue to use the new MAP with the expectation that changes will occur after longer periods of wear time. If parents observe an immediate positive change that results in improved performance, they should note these changes for the programming audiologist. This provides important feedback that can be used during subsequent mapping sessions. Some implant centers use forms and questionnaires to collect this information. (See figure 5.2.) Finally, if parents observe a negative response (either a decrease in performance or an adverse response), they should return to a previously acceptable program and contact the implant facility.

Battery Maintenance

Each implant is powered by either rechargeable or alkaline batteries. Some devices use "AA" batteries while others use lithium batteries or the traditional hearing aid button battery. Regardless, parents must be aware of the approximate life of the battery, the recharging procedure (if using rechargeable batteries), and the importance of carrying extra batteries.

Battery life varies with the type of speech processing program, the amount of wear time, and the volume settings on the processor. Certain speech processing programs require larger amounts of power. For the body processors, average battery life is approximately twelve to fifteen hours if using rechargeables, and almost twenty-four hours if using alkaline. For BTE speech processors, battery life varies greatly among devices and within a

PROGRAM DESCRIPTIONS FOR   **DATE**

PROGRAM   **DATES TO BE USED:**   -   SHAPING
map #   M levels_____   flat
                                                              mid freq emph
                                                              high freq emph
                          T levels_____   low freq emph

ENVIRONMENTAL SOUNDS: (circle all that apply)

1. No detection observed
2. Acknowledges detection of environmental sounds when directed to the sound
         within 3 feet   between 3-10 feet   at a distance > 10 feet
3. Detects environmental sounds spontaneously
         within 3 feet   between 3-10 feet   at a distance > 10 feet
4. Identifies environmental sound
         within 3 feet   between 3-10 feet   at a distance > 10 feet
5. Other, describe _____
   _____
   _____

SPEECH SOUNDS: (circle all that apply)

1. No detection observed
2. Detects Speech
         within 3 feet   between 3-10 feet   at a distance > 10 feet
3. Recognizes name
         within 3 feet   between 3-10 feet   at a distance > 10 feet
4. Recognizes isolated words
         within 3 feet   between 3-10 feet   at a distance > 10 feet
5. Recognizes common phrases
         within 3 feet   between 3-10 feet   at a distance > 10 feet
6. Other, describe _____
   _____
   _____

SPEECH PRODUCTION: (circle all that apply)

1. No detection observed
2. Increased vocalization
3. Attempts production of sounds which they previously did not attempt
4. Produces more vowels/consonants with model
5. Produces more vowels/consonants spontaneously
6. Overall intelligibility improving as indicated by better approximations of words
         (list words if possible)
7. Other, describe _____
   _____

Figure 5.2. Program Report Form

particular device. It is best to discuss the issue of battery life with the implant team.

Rechargeable batteries have to be replaced after one year of use. NiCad batteries cost substantially less than the lithium cell; however, lithium batteries recharge more quickly and hold greater power. Recharge time varies and can be as little as two hours for lithium batteries or as long as fourteen hours for NiCads. These, too, are issues to be reviewed by implant team members.

Children should carry a spare battery with them at all times. However, if the spare battery is not used for a long period of time, it will lose its charge and become nonfunctional. Also, when transporting batteries, it is best to cover the contact ends with tape or plastic; if the contact points are placed against anything metallic (such as loose change in a pocket or purse) the battery will discharge power.

Checking Microphone Function

The microphone of the cochlear implant has the same problems as hearing aid microphones. Moisture can make a microphone intermittent or completely useless. Microphone function can be assessed in a number of ways. First, the parent can do a visual inspection for any outward signs of damage or moisture. Second, the parent can ask the child to make certain auditory discriminations without the use of visual cues. (Note: this is a check that can only be performed on children who have reached a particular level of auditory sophistication.) Third, the parent can use the special plug-in microphone that comes with body-worn speech processors to see if the regular headset microphone works. By connecting this plug-in microphone with the system, the headset microphone is overridden. If the child then hears, it can be assumed that a problem exists with the headset microphone. This is an easy method of troubleshooting microphone breakdown, and the child can use the plug-in microphone until a new headset microphone can be obtained. Finally, the parent can use the microphone monitoring system that is available with some implants. Parents can listen to the microphone to make sure it is working properly. This accessory does not allow parents to listen to how the cochlear implant sounds but only to how the microphone sounds. Obviously, older children with good listening abilities will be able to report any difference in sound that may be a result of a defective microphone.

Checking the Cords

Depending on the type of implant (whether body-worn or BTE), cords connect the speech processor to the headset. In some cases, this is a two-cord system; in others, it is a one-cord system. Cords for one device will not work on another system. Parents are advised to check cords on a regular basis. Cords that are old and dried out may cause the system to go on and off. A spare set of replacement cords should be kept handy in the event they have to be changed.

Performing Daily Listening and Visual Checks of the System

Parents, teachers, and therapists working with children with cochlear implants should be comfortable handling the equipment and be able to identify signs of potential trouble. Requiring the child to perform some type of quick listening task helps parents and professionals quickly determine the overall functioning of the system. Some implant manufacturers provide a test wand that can easily be placed over the external transmitter to assess the integrity of the entire system. If the system is working, a signal on the wand lights up. Unfortunately, this test does not detect systems that may be intermittent, nor can it identify implants that are not properly tuned.

Alarms, Lights, and Icons

Some implant systems have audible alarms that signal when the battery is about to lose power, the headset has fallen off the child's head, or the cord is broken. The implant may also emit a series of light flashes or icons to indicate problems with the speech processor. These are individualized among devices. Parents should obtain the proper information from the implant center audiologist about their child's implant system.

Precautions Regarding Static Electricity

Excessive dryness can create a buildup of static electricity. Exposure to electrostatic discharge (ESD) makes the speech processor susceptible to MAP corruption. A corrupted MAP means that information on the computer chip has been altered in some way. Thus, the sound the child receives may be seriously affected or completely missing. Implant recipients or their caretakers must be aware of the precautions that need to be taken to reduce the possibility of exposure to ESD.

Plastic slides or gymnastic mats are potential sources of static electricity in the child's environment. When a child wishes to play on this equipment, parents can simply remove the external implant equipment and allow the child to play freely. Should a child play on plastic equipment while wearing the external components, there is a risk that the MAP will be erased or altered. If this happens, the parents have to take the child to the implant center so that the MAP can be rewritten to the speech processor.

Computers are another source of static electricity. To reduce the risk of ESD effects when using a computer, the child's chair should be placed on an anti-static mat and the computer should be fit with a static-proof screen. During winter months, if the classroom or home is unusually dry, it is best to spray the carpeting with an anti-static spray or a mixture that contains 50 percent water and 50 percent fabric softener. A list of these ESD precautions is available in booklet form from device manufacturers.

Precautions Regarding Moisture

In environments where the humidity is very high, external equipment may malfunction due to moisture buildup. The microphone is especially at risk since it is located either behind the ear or on the head. Individuals who perspire excessively may find that the microphone delivers an intermittent signal. Parents can prevent moisture damage through the use of a "dri-aid kit." (These same kits are used for hearing aids, too.) Parents should use these kits nightly to reduce moisture that may have built up during the day.

MRI Issues

The audiologist will outline MRI precautions during the postactivation counseling period. In order to ensure that a child is not given an MRI in an emergency, some parents choose medical alert bracelets with a "No MRI" warning. (See chapter 3 for more information about MRI compatibility issues.)

Cordless Telephones, Airports, and Security Systems

Because the implant sends its signal across the skin via FM transmission, there may, at times, be interference from other systems that operate at or near the same frequency. This may occur with some cordless telephones (those tuned to a 47-megahertz frequency). Cordless telephones in the 960-megahertz region are recommended for families with implant users to ensure that there is no disruption to the signal.

Airport security systems may detect the small amount of metal in the headset magnet and register its presence. Thus, when a child with an implant passes through the metal detector an alarm may be set off. Although identification cards are provided for implant users to present when traveling, airport personnel will likely scan the child using a hand-held wand. In some circumstances, airport security may ask the child to remove the external unit and send it through the X-ray machine. If this occurs, there is no cause for concern, as this type of inspection will not damage the implant in any way. In addition to airport metal detectors, various inventory control systems are used in libraries, department stores, and malls. Children passing through these systems will not activate the alarm but may hear a click or another type of sound.

Physical Activity

Beyond the immediate postoperative limitations on physical activity, a child with an implant can enjoy the full range of extracurricular events with the same degree of freedom as a child without an implant. Children with implants have successfully participated in hockey, horseback riding, baseball, football, soccer, skiing, and ice-skating, to name a few activities. Sports that require a helmet should be played with a helmet. Children who are involved in sports such as basketball or soccer should avoid a direct blow to the implant area. Parents may make an individual decision to limit participation in particular sporting activities simply because they do not wish to place their child at any additional risk.

Medical Precautions

Certain medical procedures are contraindicated when a child has a cochlear implant. These include diathermy and electro-convulsive shock treatments. These contraindications are outlined on the cochlear implant identification card that is provided to all recipients. The use of these treatments is very limited and does not present a real threat to the larger implant population. On the other hand, if an implant user requires any other type of surgery later in life, the implant surgeon should be contacted so that a complete medical history can be disclosed.

Contacting the Implant Center for Replacement Equipment or Other Emergencies

Regardless of how careful parents are, equipment may malfunction. When this occurs, the center should have a mechanism in place to exchange the equipment in a timely fashion. Implant facilities should outline their procedures so that there is no confusion or time wasted when a problem arises. Sometimes equipment malfunctions occur during times when the implant center is closed. Centers have different staffing availability during weekend or holiday hours. Parents should know what actions to take during these off-hours. Parents must decide what constitutes an emergency as opposed to an inconvenience. Implant manufacturers have on-call audiologists who can assist parents when contact with the implant center is not possible. Although some implant centers have on-call audiologists, most do not. Any medical emergency related to the implant should always be directed to the physician's office or on-call service immediately.

Parents are in a partnership with the implant center team to ensure that their child's implant is working appropriately each day. Parents must take this responsibility seriously since device function contributes to performance outcomes. This responsibility in the post-implant period lasts a lifetime. The implant center will do its part by assessing the child over time to monitor both external and internal device functioning. In addition, performance outcomes are assessed periodically to make certain that the implant recipient is meeting the goals suggested by the profile generated at the time of candidacy. These periodic visits will encourage continued communication with the implant center so that a child has access to the latest technological advances. Cochlear implants are a long-term commitment for both parents and children. This commitment can only be strengthened when parents and their cochlear implant team communicate on a regular basis.

Chapter 6

Learning about Listening through Home Activities

The initial switch-on of a cochlear implant is an important event; however, the real work of learning to listen begins when the child returns home after the implant is activated. At this point, an auditory focus becomes possible and, moreover, is necessary to maximize the benefits of the implant. Parents must realize that the surgeon's job has ended and the long-term work of helping their child listen with the implant has just begun. Parents who abdicate their responsibilities at home, in light of what they believe is a "medical miracle," will be disappointed with the outcome.

Many parents are thirsty for a blueprint to help their newly implanted child learn to listen; what will assist parents at this stage is a broad-based understanding of auditory skills. Determining the appropriate point at which to begin listening activities at home is dependent upon the age of the child at implantation and the level of auditory skill demonstrated prior to implant surgery. Under the dual direction of the cochlear implant center team and educational personnel, parents should be encouraged to actively participate in the habilitation of the child. In so doing, there are three important guiding principles for designing listening tasks:

1. choose the appropriate level of auditory ability,
2. select motivating activities suitable for the child's age and language ability, and
3. keep success high.

Parents or caregivers are capable of providing listening opportunities in the home and having fun with their child at the same time. In order to accomplish this goal, they must understand the stages of auditory skill development. This knowledge will enable them to become key players on the child's listening team.

It is advisable, then, that parents learn the language and vocabulary of listening skills. The terms defined in this chapter are used to describe the auditory development of children in general. An understanding of these terms will guide the parents in developing activities that are appropriate throughout the time of the child's post-implant program.

LEVELS OF AUDITORY SKILL DEVELOPMENT

☐ Detection
☐ Pattern perception
☐ Segmental identification (closed and open sets)
☐ Auditory comprehension

Detection

Detection is the most basic of all listening skills. To demonstrate this ability, a child need only indicate somehow that a sound has been heard. A child who "alerts" to a sound is demonstrating detection. Alerting to sound may take any one of a number of forms: A child engaged in an activity may cease attention to the activity and look up; an infant or toddler playing with a favorite toy will pause slightly in the activity and then continue on with play; a child may begin vocalizing when the sound occurs. For example, a child may produce a speech sound in response to the music made by a favorite toy. The observant parent will need to watch for these subtle forms of detection by a child at this level of auditory skill development and report these "sightings" to the implant center personnel.

While the alerting response is a valid means of demonstrating early detection, the child must also be taught to detect a sound in a structured activity. Active participation in evaluation tasks at the implant center (e.g., during the implant tuning or testing of the child) depends on the child's ability to demonstrate *a conditioned-response behavior*. In general, a conditioned response occurs when the child is given a stimulus (such as a sound) and learns to provide a particular response back to the examiner (such as an action). In practice, an examiner presents the child with a sound and the child demonstrates detection by raising a hand, throwing a block in a bucket, or putting a game piece on a game board. Acquisition of a conditioned response is an important task for the young child and contributes to the development and assessment of later auditory skills. Parents can help the child get ready for assessments at the implant center by taking advantage of everyday activities in the home that call for the child to wait, listen, and then respond. In this way, parents help develop the concept of a conditioned response.

The goal of the implant facility audiologist is to provide implanted children with a device set at a level that will allow them to detect sounds on the day of the initial switch-on. The age and communicative ability of each child will influence the ease with which detection will be demonstrated. Detecting sound does not imply that the sound can be identified. Regardless, parents should begin labeling the sounds in the child's environment. Parents are encouraged to take an active role in helping the child catalog his or her new world of sound. One technique for accomplishing this is to build an environmental sound dictionary.

Building the Environmental Sound Dictionary

After implantation, all children go through the process of learning to listen to the sounds that surround them. This exercise is important even for youngsters who had listening experience through hearing aids. Sound processed by the implant is different from sound delivered through hearing aids. Parental involvement is crucial in building the environmental sound dictionary in the home. As parents observe a child alert to a sound, especially an environmental sound, they can label and describe it. For children who use a form of manual communication, this label and description can be presented in sign. Keep in mind that there are hundreds of sounds in our homes—not just the obvious ones (the telephone, the microwave timer, and the doorbell), but also sounds that hearing individuals have grown accustomed to over time and tend to ignore. Household noises, such as the refrigerator, heating and cooling systems, and even loud ticking clocks, may turn parents into "sound detectives" searching for a particular sound source.

It is likely that a child will need numerous listening and labeling opportunities before these acoustical events become permanent entries in the environmental sound dictionary and before they can be identified independently. Parents are urged to refrain from testing the child during this period. Labeling the sound that has been detected and describing its characteristics are the key charges to parents of children at this stage of auditory skill. For example, if the child alerts to the sound of running water as the dishwasher fills, the parent can call attention to the sound and give more descriptors of it (either verbally or through sign): "That's the water coming into the dishwasher; it is a sound that goes on for a while and then stops."

Setting a Listening Window

When building the environmental sound dictionary, it can be helpful to set a "listening window" for the child. When the parent knows that a sound is about to occur, the parent describes it first and then encourages the child to wait and listen for it. Upon hearing the target sound, the child responds in some way indicating that it has been detected. Setting a listening window could be as simple as waiting for the microwave timer to beep while dinner is being cooked. Parents can also announce that a visitor will soon arrive at the house and will ring the doorbell before entering. When the child hears the doorbell, he or she can go and greet the guest.

Setting a listening window relieves the child of the burden of constantly scanning the auditory environment in anticipation of sounds that are about to occur. Focusing attention to the listening task will prevent the child from being distracted from other events or activities that are occurring. The task of detection is made easier when the parent prepares the child ahead of time to listen.

Creating Opportunities for Building Speech Detection Skills

For the very young child or the child who has yet to develop the conditioned response task, parents may have to provide particular listening opportunities for detecting speech. It is especially important to imbed meaningful detection opportunities in age-appropriate and motivating play activities. As with any listening activity, the need to make the task *auditory-only* is an essential element. This principle becomes even more important for children who communicate with sign. Many individuals, parents and teachers alike, are momentarily uncomfortable with the idea of withholding sign and other visual information from deaf children. However, a task is not auditory unless all visual clues are removed.

The "formula" for all listening tasks is quite fundamental and is something that all parents can learn, regardless of their child's level of auditory skill. The series of steps is as follows:

1. the parent says a word, phrase, or sentence that the child cannot see,
2. the child listens to what the parent says, and
3. the child indicates, in some way, that speech has been heard.

The parent can make this task more or less difficult by altering what is said and changing the response demands of the child. The constant element in an auditory exercise is that the child *only listens* to what the parent says. This can be accomplished in one of several ways. The most natural approach to making a task auditory is for the parent to sit beside or behind the child when speaking. From either of these locations, the child is unable to see the parent's mouth for cues from facial expressions or speechreading. Young children are accustomed to being held on a parent's lap during story time. (A special section devoted to listening with books will be found later in this chapter.)

Learning to Wait

When the focus of a listening activity is detection, it does not matter *what* is said, only that the child waits and responds to speech appropriate to the event. The word or phrase should be familiar to the child and should make sense in the context of the activity. The parent tells the child what to listen for and begins the game. Any toy manipulation activity can be used to practice learning to wait. For example, in the game in which smaller barrels are housed inside larger barrels, the child delays opening the barrel until mom says "open." The child knows that the word "open" will serve as the target; the critical component in a detection task is the wait time until the parent actually says the word. Young children have a difficult time waiting in general. Asking them to wait until they hear something requires additional discipline. It is important, however, that a child understands and follows the rules of the listening game. Otherwise, it will be difficult to determine if the child is learning the task of speech detection. The child should not respond before or at the same time the parent speaks. If this occurs, it is likely that the child did not understand the waiting portion of the detection task and needs further practice. Parents interested in creating detection tasks will find a wealth of materials right inside their child's toy box. In addition, everyday parent–child activities such as dressing or getting ready for dinner can also lend themselves easily to developing detection skills.

When a Child Detects and Recognizes His or Her Name

The greatest reward in the early days of implant use occurs when the child recognizes his or her own name. One way to achieve this is to play turn-taking activities in which the child waits to hear his or her name before completing an action—perhaps marking a paper with a rubber stamp in different color inks. With repeated exposure in detection tasks, children learn the sound of their own name.

As auditory skill develops, the child may begin to recognize his or her name in natural settings. Parents of hearing children take for granted the meaning of this small auditory task. Many parents of implanted children have reported that this accomplishment was their single most important goal. Parents of children with significant hearing loss are often unable to get their child's attention from beyond the visual (or perhaps tactile) field. In the daily management of the household, the physical task of gaining the child's attention often interrupts the flow of everyday events. The ability of a child with an implant to recognize his or her name being called from another room is a skill highly valued by most parents. For older children, the ability to hear their name from behind a closed door may afford them the privacy that previously eluded them.

Moving through the Stage of Speech and Environmental Sound Detection

The rate at which any individual child moves through a stage of auditory skill development varies widely. However, detection of speech and environmental sounds is the entry-level stage of auditory skill development. Most children will likely pass through

73

this stage in a timely fashion that is related to their chronological age. Older children will pass through this phase more quickly than one- or two-year-olds; cognitive development and the ability to participate in the conditioned response task will speed the journey of the newly implanted child who is older. On the other hand, individuals continue to refine their skills within a particular stage even after they have entered the next phase of skill development. This may be true even of the entry-level stage of detection. As a child continues to refine detection skills, he or she may hear sounds previously judged by parents to be too soft (such as chirping birds). Parents should not overlook even the quietest sounds in the environment when the child demonstrates awareness of them.

Sometimes a child will need added practice to carry over detection easily demonstrated in a quiet environment to an environment that is filled with everyday noise. Furthermore, a child may get used to certain sounds in the environment and, after a while, no longer alert to them. Hearing people do this all the time; it follows then, that children with implants may also ignore environmental sounds once the novelty of alerting to particular sounds has worn off. Parents should not be alarmed if previously demonstrated detection skills seem to be lost. This is especially true if the child progresses to the next phase of auditory skill development, pattern perception.

Pattern Perception

A child is ready for the next stage of listening skill, *pattern perception*, when he or she shows consistent detection of sound in both quiet and natural environments. Pattern perception builds on detection and takes the listening task to a higher level. The ability to tell long from short sounds or continuous from interrupted signals indicates pattern recognition for environmental sounds. A child who can differentiate between a car horn honking (short, interrupted sounds) and the noise made by a lawnmower (a continuous and long sound) is demonstrating pattern recognition. Similarly, being able to tell a long sentence from a short sentence ("Let's read a book before bed" vs. "Brush your teeth") is a demonstration of pattern perception. The ability to perceive patterns can also be demonstrated at the word level, for example, by distinguishing between a three-syllable word and a one-syllable word (banana vs. pear).

Identifying the Elements of Pattern Perception Tasks

In order to design a pattern perception activity that is auditory-only, there must be at least two stimuli or choices that are known to the child, and they must differ somehow in the patterns. These activities start with a set of choices called a *closed set*. This means that all the possible answers are known before listening begins. The parent says one of the words in the closed set without the child looking. The child must then choose the correct word based only on the pattern of the speech or sound. For purposes of clarification, examples of selected activities and the closed sets appropriate to them are detailed below.

A typical play activity can be used to practice differentiating between words that have several syllables and words that have only one syllable. When a mother and daughter play dress-up bear, this interaction provides opportunities to create closed set listening tasks. First, and most importantly, mom labels all items of clothing in the set. She must choose two items of clothing that have different syllable lengths to form the first closed set (hat vs. purple dress). These items become the closed set from which the child will select the word he or she hears. If the mother and child use sign language as their primary communication mode, then directions for this activity should be given using both sign and speech. However, the activity itself must be presented in an auditory-only mode. In this activity of pattern perception, it is not necessary for the child to understand and hear clearly the exact words *hat* or *purple dress*; she is listening only for something short vs. something long. Mom sits beside the girl so she cannot see her mouth and presents the *stimulus* word, "hat." In this scenario, the daughter's *response* is choosing the correct item of clothing from the set of two and then dressing the bear. Other items of clothing can be used to form additional closed sets, reinforce new vocabulary, and provide the child with more listening opportunities. This naturalistic activity practices listening in a way that is age-appropriate, fun, and motivating for the child.

Parameters of Pattern Perception Tasks

For the skill of pattern perception to develop to its fullest, the number of items in the set should increase as the child becomes more skilled. Thus, in the situation outlined above, one method of making the task more difficult would be to include a third item in the closed set (add *black purse* to the choices *purple dress* and *hat*). Increasing the size of the set requires that each word pattern in the set be different from the others. If a pattern perception task is too difficult, it is necessary to decrease the size of the closed set. (Keep in mind, however, that there must be at least two items in the set since the child needs to make a choice.)

The Ongoing Stage of Pattern Perception

The skill of pattern perception should be reviewed and reinforced each time the child encounters new vocabulary. When a child learns new words as part of experiential and language development, the established skill of pattern perception can be practiced. At the same time, listening skills are reinforced. For example, a child who is learning new vocabulary in the area of transportation may encounter words such as *jeep* and *ambulance*.

One should immediately see that the first new word has one syllable and the second has three syllables. Observant parents can seize this opportunity to practice listening skills. These new words create a listening experience for the child. For example, while playing with the jeep and ambulance, the parent can provide this listening prompt, "Here comes something down the road. It's the *ambulance*!" Upon hearing the multisyllable target instead of the single-syllable target, the child picks up the ambulance and "drives" it down the road. Once again, a naturalistic play activity provides the material for a quick listening task.

The Role of Speech in Listening Activities

Both of the examples of pattern perception activities just described require the child to respond by performing an action. While this is a perfectly acceptable response to the pattern perception task, parents should not overlook the importance of getting the child to use his or her newfound hearing ability to produce speech. Listening and speaking complement one another. Children who can hear use this sense to learn speech. The cochlear implant enables a child to have access to the sounds that make up everyday spoken language. Thus, the cochlear implant is not only a listening tool, it is a speaking tool as well.

Activities that do not include any type of spoken response can seriously limit improvements in speech skills. The simplest way to encourage the child to practice speech skills during a listening game is to let the child take a turn as the speaker, while the parent becomes the listener. The child's speech need not be perfect, but it should be clear enough to communicate the key information that will allow the adult to respond correctly. In the example above, the child who wants to give the stimulus *jeep* should produce only one syllable and attempt to match the vowel sound of the word if possible. A proper production of the /j/ sound is not necessary at this level for some children.

Segmental Identification (Closed and Open Sets)

The stage of listening skill development immediately following pattern perception is *segmental identification.* In segmental identification, a child no longer relies on patterns to differentiate words but uses information from the speech sounds of the words to identify the target. Words, phrases, and sentences at this level all have the same patterns. When the words, phrases, and sentences have the same patterns, the child is required to listen more closely to other speech features to recognize them. This stage encompasses a large number of subskills, and it is likely that a child will spend a significant period of time moving through this important phase of auditory skill development.

Closed Sets and Segmental Identification

At the very start of segmental identification work, small closed sets of all the possible choices are presented to the child. For segmental identification tasks, the makeup of the words (phrases or sentences) in the closed set is critical. A good closed set for a beginning listener will have two or three items, and the items themselves will not have the same sounds in them. For example, a closed set that has the items *rabbit, turtle,* and *lion* is better than a closed set that has *monkey, donkey,* and *giraffe* or *chicken, kitten,* and *piglet.* Initially, parents should avoid using rhyming words or those with the same vowel sounds. Notice that in the first closed set, all three items have the same number of syllables but the sounds of the words are very different. There is a short "a" sound in *rabbit, turtle* has a strong "ur" in it, and the word *lion* has the long "i" sound. In contrast, each of the next two closed sets presents a problem to the beginning listener. In the set *donkey, monkey,* and *giraffe,* the first two words are very similar. Posing this closed set to a listener just beginning the segmental identification task may make it too difficult. In the final example (*chicken, kitten, piglet*), all of the items in the closed set have both a short "i" sound in the first syllable and a short "e" sound in the second syllable. This closed set is quite challenging and would be appropriate for a child with more advanced segmental identification skills. Only an experienced listener would be able to choose confidently from a set containing items that are so closely linked. Remarkably, the ability to make this kind of distinction is well within the reach of children who use cochlear implants over an extended period of time.

Thus far, all of the sets examined contain only three items. In order to challenge children who are successful with small closed sets, the size of the set should increase over time. In segmental identification, a skilled listener may have many items in a closed set task—perhaps eight or more. The basic rule for designing closed sets for segmental identification tasks is as follows:

If the child is having success, increase the size of the set and/or use words with more similar sounds; if the child is having difficulty, decrease the number of items in the set and/or make the items in the set more different.

The child's level of success or difficulty will lead the parent or caregiver in the right direction for creating closed set tasks at this level. Parents should remember that it is easy to incorporate listening activities into the daily routine of the home. The items in the closed set can be common objects around the kitchen, the living room, the family room, or the child's bedroom. For example, in the kitchen, while setting the table for dinner, ask the child to "put the _____ (*knife, fork,* or *spoon*)" on the table; while getting dressed, tell the child to "put on _____ (*socks, pants,* or *shirt*)."

Level of Language Input

The listening activities described thus far are natural and capitalize on the child's interests. These examples use individual words as the listening targets. However, it is also important for the child to learn to attend to more than just one word at a time. Sentences, at this stage, must all have the same patterns so that true segmental identification ability is practiced. Using activities that occur in any household, parents can structure sentences that highlight segmental identification tasks. For example, following a conversation about favorite TV shows, a closed set of target sentences can be developed for a listening activity later in the day.

1. My favorite show is *Arthur*.
2. Dad's favorite show is *E.R.*
3. Mom's favorite show is *Oprah*.
4. Gran's favorite show is the news.

All of these sentences follow the same pattern, so the child has to rely on the segmental information to differentiate between and among the sentences. Once the child is successful with a particular closed set, additional sentences can be added to make the task more challenging. Again, it is extremely important that listening activities provide an opportunity for speaking. All too often, parents and even therapists will challenge the child's listening abilities without encouraging speaking skills. For this reason, the child should always be given the opportunity to repeat the word or sentence and to present the listening stimulus in this guessing game activity.

Bridging to Open Set Tasks

In contrast to closed set tasks, open set tasks require the child to listen to a stimulus that has not been previously identified. In fact, in an open set task, the listening choices are endless. This level of speech recognition is the gold standard in listening ability for children and adults with implants. In order to reach this goal, the child is often provided with "bridge" sets. These are sets in which the child knows the topic or category, which limits the choices; however, the exact items presented are not known. Parents may begin this guessing game by telling the child, "I'm going to name some clothes." Then the adult, using a listening-only presentation, names articles of clothing for the child to repeat (*belt, shoes, jacket, t-shirt*). In this game, the child's clear production of speech is especially important. When it is the child's turn to name the category and be responsible for giving each individual stimulus, intelligible speech is mandatory to make the game possible.

Auditory Comprehension

The final developmental stage of listening is *auditory comprehension*. At this level, rather than simply repeating what was said, a child answers a question or responds in some way that is different from the stimulus. For example, a child who correctly answers the question, "What is the name of your school?" (after the question has been posed through listening only), is demonstrating auditory comprehension. One technique that appears to be natural for this skill level is the "opposite game." Here the parent says a word such as *dirty,* and the child responds correctly with *clean.* In order to be successful in this game, of course, the child must understand the concept of opposites and must possess an appropriate vocabulary.

As children mature, parents can make the listening task more challenging by posing riddles that have multiple parts. In this instance, a parent may provide the following clues: "I'm thinking of an animal you can see at the zoo. It looks a little like a horse. It has black and white stripes." With these clues, a child should be able to name the animal *zebra*, thereby demonstrating auditory comprehension.

For the older child with an implant, homework assignments, spelling activities, and math facts practice can be successfully used to sharpen auditory comprehension skills. When working with teenagers, more motivating topics or activities can be used; school-based activities need not be used. The simple art of conversation requires a strong component of auditory comprehension. Therefore, exchanges related to sports, clothing, music, and special events lend themselves well to these types of listening challenges.

Book Reading and Other Familiar Parent–Child Activities

The everyday activities associated with managing the household have been recommended as a good place to start to engage the child in listening. However, it is important not to overlook the auditory activities that normally occur for young children everywhere: book reading, nursery rhymes, and finger-play. These, too, provide an excellent opportunity for the child with an implant to listen to the language of the home in a manner that is pleasurable and age-appropriate. There is, perhaps, no greater comfort to a young child than being held lovingly by a parent or caregiver. Adding an auditory component to a postfeeding or bedtime ritual by singing a lullaby or sharing a folksong provides an infant with an enriched listening opportunity.

Parents do not always have to design an activity that presents a target stimulus or prompts a correct response. Many naturally occurring parent–child interactions already set listening as a priority. Recall the songs of your own childhood and be sure to share them with your child. This listening activity offers a playful experience and provides an opportunity to pass along the culture or heritage of the family, which is especially important when members of the immediate or extended family speak another language. There is no better opportunity to capitalize on the grandparents' role and include them in the post-implant habilitative process.

Experts in the field of reading have long encouraged parents to begin literacy activities with their children as early as possible. For deaf children with implants, the initial reading of a book might be a face-to-face instructional activity as the child learns the characters and/or the actions of the book. Later readings (and there may be hundreds for favorite books) can lend themselves, in a number of ways, to listening-only activities. As noted earlier, the shared book-reading activity allows for auditory-only input because the child is seated on the reader's lap, facing forward, away from the reader. Other book-reading auditory activities may include:

- listening for the parent's voice to stop so the child will know when to turn the page,
- saying the last word on the page (this is done by memory, as a precursor to true reading),
- pointing to items or objects illustrated on the page as they are named by the parent (don't overdo this as it takes away from the concept of the story as a whole), and
- answering questions about what will happen next in the story.

All of the listening levels described earlier can be found in these suggested strategies. Children at all stages of listening development can benefit from shared book-reading activities with parents, caregivers, grandparents, and even siblings. The natural tasks associated with reading to a child are among the best auditory activities to motivate and hold the interest of young children.

The Power of the Parent at Home

Parents should not underestimate the effect they have on their children's listening lives. Implant centers recognize this role and ask that parents become partners in the post-implant habilitation process. The home represents the most familiar surrounding for the child and serves as the first classroom. Participating in family life brings with it a multitude of opportunities for a child to expand auditory knowledge. Parents do not have to be "trained" teachers, but, by being a focused parent and seizing the "teachable" moment, they can profoundly influence their child's overall auditory development.

Chapter 7

The Cochlear Implant as a Tool for Language Development

All parents want to be able to communicate with their children and have them communicate back. When a child is born, parents wait anxiously for their baby's first word. If spoken language is the language of the home, hearing parents of deaf children are even more anxious since the hearing loss may seriously delay this important milestone. Choosing a communication modality, then, is critically important as hearing parents begin to make decisions regarding their deaf child. For some parents the choice is easy; others agonize over making the "right" decision. There is no crystal ball that allows parents to see into the future of any child. Parents who are paralyzed about making choices often lose valuable time that sometimes compromises the end result. Yet, parents should not make decisions for the sake of decision-making, especially without considering information that can assist them in the process. No parent ever willfully makes a choice that is believed to be a poor one. Parents cannot immediately see the outcome of many of their decisions, but they make them in good faith and in the best interests of the child.

Hearing parents of deaf children face the ultimate dilemma: Does the family learn an entirely new way to communicate (sign language), or do they facilitate the child's learning of the spoken language of the home? When the latter choice is made, parents are already experts in that language. In the former case, parents must become proficient, in a short period of time, in a language for which they have no prior knowledge and limited exposure to expert users. If parents choose a manual language, then, in order to provide the richest linguistic environment for their child, they must learn it themselves. Children use language to learn about their world and subsequently learn more about language through their world. Thus, it is imperative to make a commitment to develop good language regardless of its nature and form.

Greater numbers of hearing parents are choosing implantation for their children because it provides them with the opportunity to communicate using their native spoken language. However, many parents view sign language as an important part of their deaf child's development. Numerous families have successfully integrated spoken communication with sign language. Whether parents choose the manual or the oral approach, the important issue is that the communication method chosen provide the necessary input for language development. A cochlear implant assists in this task.

When cochlear implants first appeared on the technological scene, they were reserved for adults and viewed as a device that would improve speech perception (listening to and understanding speech). For late-deafened adults, improvements in speech perception seemed a reasonable expectation. An added benefit for many of these individuals included changes in speech clarity. The technology delivered the sounds of the language and provided access to better vocal monitoring, thereby enabling these deaf adults to listen to themselves and speak more clearly. It was anticipated that when implants were placed in children, they would have a similar effect. Years later, when implants were first investigated in the pediatric population, the following questions emerged about benefits to both speech perception and speech production:

- Could the implant provide more than an opportunity to hear sounds and talk more clearly?
- How would the implant actually help congenitally deaf or prelinguistically deafened children?

After more than a decade of research on the implantation of young deaf children, we now know that increased access to sound through a cochlear implant benefits speech perception, speech production, and even the development of spoken English. A closer look at language learning may shed some light on the relationship between the cochlear implant and the acquisition of English.

English as an Auditory Oral Language

The English language, like most of the languages of the world, is an auditory, oral language. Despite the fact that it has a written form that can be accessed visually, the language is designed to be heard and spoken. Because of this auditory component, a great number of deaf children have had difficulty learning English. Published research documenting the English language abilities of deaf children reveals that many of the more complex forms of English syntax are absent or only partially present. In addition, deaf children have impoverished vocabularies, with both a smaller number of words and minimal variety.

What accounts for this disappointing language-learning performance? Most obviously, learning a spoken language is a difficult task for youngsters with significant hearing loss since they are unable to access critical portions of the speech signal. Deaf children in strictly oral programs have been asked to learn spoken English through a sensory system that is not fully functional despite the best-fit hearing aids. Deaf children in programs that present manual codes of English (such as Signed English or Signing Exact English) have been asked to process an auditory/oral language visually. Thus, in both oral and sign language programs, the natural process of learning this spoken language called English is impeded.

Cochlear implant technology decreases the first barrier, the access barrier, to learning spoken English. The implant provides auditory information that makes the process of learning English easier. It improves the delivery of the sounds of English so that it can be learned in its natural state, as an auditory/oral language. While some deaf children have successfully learned English through visual representations of English and reading and writing, they are alternate, rather than primary, routes. If English is the language of your home and/or the development of English is an educational goal for your deaf child, cochlear implant technology provides the *most direct avenue* for accessing the English language. For large numbers of early implanted deaf children, English develops in a manner more similar to that of hearing children than profoundly deaf children using hearing aids and/or sign communication. This means that parents can take a more naturalistic approach to communicating with their deaf child and subsequently foster language learning.

Learning Language

It is well documented that languages are not *taught* to young children, rather, children *learn* language through everyday use in meaningful contexts at home and in play. The greater the similarity between the parents' natural language and the child's access to that language, the greater the likelihood that language will develop according to predetermined milestones. Hearing children of hearing parents *and* deaf children of deaf parents are perfect examples of this phenomenon at work. Obviously, hearing children of hearing parents have easy access to language models that utilize auditory and spoken signals. Because American Sign Language (ASL) is a visual language and because deaf children have unimpaired access to information presented visually, their development of ASL parallels the development of auditory-oral language in hearing youngsters. Cochlear implants, especially when provided to infants, allow deaf children of hearing parents (learning English) to approach language parity with deaf children of deaf parents (learning ASL). When hearing parents of deaf children choose implantation, parents use their natural language and the child has greater access to it.

Homes with Spoken Languages Other Than English

What if English is not the language of the home? Perhaps the home language is Spanish, Korean, Polish, or Urdu. There is nothing specific to English that makes it the only language that can be processed through a cochlear implant. Cochlear implants are available worldwide and children are successful regardless of their country of origin. In fact, cochlear implants enable foreign-born parents of profoundly deaf children to share an important part of their home culture with their child—their native language. Because the home language of hearing parents of foreign birth is a spoken language and because the implant delivers the signals of all spoken languages, parents can use their native language with the assurance that the child can hear it. However, these children are likely to be enrolled in an English-based school program, thus creating a second language input. For this reason, there may be a delay in the emergence of both languages. Some implant programs discourage the use of a second language in the home because they fear that it will impede the acquisition of English. Other programs acknowledge the presence of the home language and the richness of the cultural experience it offers to the young child. At the present time, there is no research to support either position. It is hoped that future research will address this issue.

Signs or Manual Codes of English for Language Learning

Some parents who choose implantation for their child have already made the decision to include sign as a part of their overall communication plan. These parents, committed to capitalizing on a deaf infant's early reliance on visual information, utilize sign communication for early language development while investigating implantation. In fact, there appears to be a growing movement to support introduction of sign for *all* infants, deaf and hearing. Recent research documents the appearance of recognizable signs before a child is able to produce a spoken first word since the child is capable of the gross motor movements of the hands before the finer motor movements of speech. Many parents who sign during the pre-implant stage have, as their long-term goal, a plan for the child to transition to spoken English as the primary means of communication. They expect that the child will use spoken English exclusively for both receptive and expressive language development.

Another group of parents will continue to sign with their children even after implantation. These parents view the implant as a tool that is added to their primary communication plan of lifelong sign language usage. Unfortunately, there may be some implant center teams that will disapprove of the use of sign language after implant surgery. Parents who are committed to the use of sign for language learning and communication should know that there are also a large number of implant centers that will support the parents' choice. In these centers, post-implant habilitation programs are tailored to the individual child and respect and support the communication goals that the parents have chosen.

At this juncture, it is necessary to introduce and clarify two terms that are used and often misused regarding the issue of communicating via sign language. The term *Total Communication* (TC) has been used colloquially to identify the philosophy of schools and programs that are not oral but use sign in conjunction with speech. The original meaning assigned to this term suggested that schools practicing "total" communication provided the communication system appropriate to the child's needs from the continuum of communication options. Thus, one child would have access to ASL, whereas another might use oral communication. The more precise term *Simultaneous*

Communication refers to the practice of talking and signing at the same time. Most cochlear implant recipients who use sign are educated in these Simultaneous Communication environments, although the more commonly abbreviated TC may be used to designate that the program is not an oral-only program. *Parents must be clear about the distinction and determine how any school or program identifies itself and how that school chooses to define the label in use.*

ASL as a Home Language

ASL is a visual spatial language used largely by deaf individuals to communicate without voice. Presently, there are only a small number of children who use ASL at home *and* who use the implant to process spoken English. Until now, few members of the Deaf community have sought implantation for their children since it was not believed to contribute substantially to their cultural persona. In fact, the vast majority of Deaf community members have been resistant to implantation in children. This opposition from the Deaf community is woven into a complex fabric of historic, linguistic, political, and educational factors that is difficult for persons with a hearing worldview to fully appreciate. It is an unusual circumstance for a deaf family using ASL as the home language to choose implantation for their child. Insight into this issue has recently been offered through an acclaimed documentary entitled *Sound and Fury*. In the rare cases when deaf parents using ASL choose implantation for their child, they do so to assist the child in functioning within the larger hearing community.

When a child's home language is ASL, a substantial portion of the responsibility to provide spoken language input falls to the school program. When the child attends a public school, this responsibility is fairly easy to fulfill. The child is exposed to hearing teachers and hearing students throughout the school day. However, the situation is very different in a school for deaf children. Some of these schools have developed bilingual/bicultural programs that use ASL as the primary language of instruction and provide access to English only in its written form. If the implant is to provide any benefit at all, there must be spoken language to process throughout the child's day. But like two forms of matter, ASL and spoken English cannot occupy the same space at the same time. Schools for deaf students continue to debate their role in service delivery to children with implants from either deaf or hearing families. Some schools using ASL are now considering spoken-language classrooms for their children with implants so that they can add an enriched language experience to the existing rich cultural environment. Educators are keeping a close watch on these programs to learn more about providing instruction to children with implants in schools that have designated ASL as their primary language of instruction.

Cued Speech

Another communication tool that is available to children with hearing loss and their parents is Cued Speech. Cued Speech should not be mistaken as a sign system or a language; it is a set of hand symbols to support the recognition of spoken English through speechreading. Based on the premise that the many English speech sounds look alike on the lips, Cued Speech supplements the limited auditory clues and confusing visual speechreading movements with a hand symbol that identifies exactly the sounds of spoken language. This complex method is a closed system, and a motivated parent could learn the basics of this communication tool in a short period of time. When a child using Cued Speech becomes a candidate for implantation, best practice dictates that the child continue the use of this system after implantation. Research suggests that as auditory experience with the implant increases, the child's reliance upon secondary support systems such as Cued Speech decreases.

Using the Cochlear Implant for Language Learning

Regardless of whether or not sign is used as a tool for language learning, once a child receives a cochlear implant, a new avenue for processing language is available. When children with mild to moderate forms of hearing loss have appropriate amplification from their hearing aids, they are capable of developing language systems that are on a par with hearing language learners. Profoundly deaf children who use cochlear implants have the potential to be more like children with a lesser degree of hearing loss who use their residual hearing to gain access to the speech signal. With this in mind, several principles can guide parents in their journey toward helping their implanted child develop spoken language.

Principle 1. There Is a Unique Relationship between Listening and Language

Children who hear speech either with or without amplification are capable of decoding it to learn spoken language. The amount of effort that is required by any individual child depends on his or her level of hearing as well as the integrity of the language-learning system in the brain. Some children with intact hearing may still need help to focus on listening to the sounds of the language in order to acquire proficiency. Likewise, children with hearing loss can benefit from enhanced listening opportunities by using their sense of hearing to learn language. Parents who provide children with enriched auditory experiences from early infancy ensure that the contributions of audition to language learning can be maximized.

Language is "bootstrapped" onto the listening skills of the child who is implanted soon after the first year of life. The implant provides deaf infants with the potential for an auditory experience that is similar to the one that drives language learning for children without hearing loss. Thus, the implanted child learns to listen to extract language and uses language to learn more about listening. When implantation occurs at the end of or beyond the critical language-learning years, the process is often reversed. The child enters implantation with an established level of language skill that is then used to develop listening ability. Parents who use the child's established language skills to sharpen listening behaviors find that, with experience, these sharpened listening behaviors contribute to further language development.

Principle 2. The World Is a Place To Be Narrated

Parents who continually narrate and offer "color commentary" of their world provide the language of the external experiences to match the internal prelinguistic representations their children have developed. To ensure explicit language learning, the best narrations for young children are those that focus on people and events in the "here and now." Mutual gaze between parents and infants is a precursor to on-topic "conversations." Mothers often use these brief eye contacts with their infants to comment upon the activity or object that is within the immediate visual environment. In this manner, children learn that objects have names and that these names and the objects they stand for are constant. This is not beyond the normal parent–child communication paradigm and should be continued for children who use implants.

Principle 3. Every Opportunity for Listening Is an Opportunity for Speaking.

The earliest language behaviors to appear include labeling, getting needs and wants met, and commenting on the environment. These begin as gestures, mature to vocalizations, and eventually become recognizable words. Parents who prompt their children to respond to communication or react to events with speech reinforce the auditory/speech feedback loop. In so doing, they set an expectation for a spoken response and a precedent for how to participate in communication exchanges. If parents do not encourage a child to generate speech on a regular basis, the skills required to produce spoken language have limited opportunity to develop. Parents must walk a fine line, however, when prompting speech from their child. It is important to understand that speech cannot be forced from a child. Parents will want to help the child see speech as a source of power, not as a burden in communication exchanges.

Principle 4. Language Growth Occurs through Exchanges with a Mature Language User

Models of language development presume that the language learner is exposed to a sophisticated language expert. The language expert identifies the level of language of the novice user and develops it to the next level. When a child acknowledges an airplane passing overhead by pointing and/or saying "airplane," the language expert expands this label and may add, "The airplane is going fast." This technique, known as expansion, recasts the child's utterances into an enriched linguistic unit that is just beyond the child's present functioning. Recasts may add new vocabulary, modify labels, or introduce more complex sentence structure. The technique of expansion suggests that when children hear the new language, it eventually is added into their language repertoire.

These four principles are, by no means, exhaustive in scope; however, they are the basis from which language facilitation can evolve. Parents who choose an oral approach will provide input using spoken language exclusively. Parents who use a sign system for their language activities will follow a similar blueprint but must be careful to provide auditory input and extract speech from the child when appropriate.

Communication choices for deaf children with implants are the same as those for deaf children who do not use implants. Choosing a particular approach is no guarantee that a child will succeed in that approach. Parents who are knowledgeable of the continuum of communication options that exist for their child recognize that movement between and among these options may occur as their child's language-learning needs change. Children's social and emotional needs may also influence modality preference as they accommodate to ever-changing communication environments.

Chapter 8

School Placement Issues

The education of deaf children has long been a topic of great controversy. The basic argument revolves around *how* a deaf child should be educated: orally or using a form of manual communication. These options were outlined in the previous chapter from the perspective of a family making a communication choice after the initial identification of hearing loss. Oftentimes, schools and programs for deaf children align themselves with particular philosophies. Professionals in the field of deaf education have, within their lifetime, seen movement from one end of the communication continuum to the other. Proponents of each philosophy have touted the success of its stars and have urged adoption of that strategy for all deaf children. It is now generally accepted that there is no one way that all deaf children should communicate and that a host of factors contribute to the parents' decision about a communication mode for their individual child.

The first decision that parents have to make for their deaf child is to select a communication modality. Unfortunately, this important decision must be made as soon as possible so that the parents can begin the natural process of communicating with their child. For parents of a very young, newly identified deaf child, the next decision, the decision of *where* the deaf child is to be educated does not present itself until somewhat later. As the child approaches the age of three and reaches the end of eligibility for Early Intervention services, the parent is offered educational options from which to choose. Today's choices vary significantly and have grown out of both social and legislative movements. A closer look at how events and circumstances of the past have shaped current educational placement options may prove helpful.

A Historical Perspective on Educational Placement Choice

Before the passage of the landmark legislation known as Public Law (PL) 94-142 (the Education for All Handicapped Children Act, now known as IDEA—Individuals with Disabilities Education Act) in 1975, the question of where a deaf child was to be educated was rarely asked. Prior to that legislation, parents essentially had two options—a day or residential school for deaf children, either publicly or privately run, or public school. It should be noted that, prior to 1975, public school services were often reserved for only high-achieving, orally educated deaf students. At that time, there were virtually no support systems in place for students with special needs in regular school programs. Those children who were successful in class received no services through the school and relied upon parental or private outside help. After the passage of PL 94-142, however, services for all children with learning differences improved markedly. For deaf children, this resulted in an increased number of educational placements in the public schools and in regional day programs.

Regional Schools for Deaf Children

Regional schools or programs for deaf children were generally formed when a number of communities joined together to develop services for students with hearing loss. Each participating community contributed to the pool of monies used to finance the program. Deaf children from various towns traveled to a central location where education and support services were clustered. A regional program could be housed in a stand-alone facility or could operate in a section of a neighborhood school.

Educational services for deaf children were centralized for a number of reasons. First, since the occurrence of deafness in the general population is relatively low, an individual town might not have enough children to form a class. Bringing children from several communities together enabled school districts to create a critical mass from which class-sized groups could be organized to provide appropriate instruction. Regionalization of programs also allowed for the sharing of instructional costs and the expense of related support required by deaf children. These included audiology, speech, language, and interpreter services as well as amplification equipment. One of the negative aspects associated with these regionalized programs for deaf children was the travel time required for many of the students. In heavily congested areas, traffic volume was a problem; in rural areas, sheer distance to the center accounted for the long travel time.

Day Classes for Deaf Children

When individual communities had a sufficient number of students to make a class of their own, day classes for deaf children were established and housed in neighborhood schools. Instructional groups were formed, and children received academic services from trained teachers of deaf children. Since deaf students then attended the same school as hearing students, "social mainstreaming" was possible in this setting. Social mainstreaming is generally defined as an opportunity for all students to participate in the nonacademic portions of the school day: lunch, recess, gym, and art. Once one municipality established day classes, neighboring communities could send their deaf students to that program as an out-of-district, tuition-paying pupil. Some school districts were committed to providing day classes for children with hearing loss within their general education program and have continued to do so despite the fact that no child enrolled in the program is a resident of that community.

Inclusion

The philosophy of inclusion is based on the belief that a student's primary point of service delivery is in the general education classroom. Special technology and/or support personnel are brought into the classroom to enable the child with special needs to be successful in that environment. Oftentimes, inclusionary practices call for additional staff in the classroom with the regular education teacher. This individual may be a certified teacher, an instructional assistant, or a personal aide. Inclusion, which has its roots in the reauthorization of IDEA in 1997, is often mislabeled, frequently overused, and largely misunderstood by parents (not to mention some educators and administrators). This educational approach is opposed by many in the deafness field as being inappropriate for students with hearing loss. Some educators and administrators fear that schools will corral deaf students into regular classes based on bottom-line finances rather than the abilities and needs of the students. As the larger special education community moves forward to embrace inclusion, parents of deaf children should be aware of the premise behind it and be able to recognize good practices. As educational advocates for their children, parents should also be wary of inclusion that is poorly implemented.

Generally speaking, included students have sufficient language and academic skills to access the regular curriculum. However, modifications in the amount of material covered and the ways in which the material is presented are often made. It follows then, that the greater the number of changes in the scope and delivery of the regular curriculum, the more specialized the person responsible for adapting and delivering the modifications must be. For example, a second-grade *included* student will receive instruction under the dual direction of a general education teacher *and* a teacher of deaf children. The teacher of deaf children selects the content and modifies the instruction and assignments as needed to parallel the regular second-grade curriculum. In some cases, interpreters are also a part of the inclusion team.

Mainstreaming

After PL 94-142, mainstreaming continued to be available to students with the academic skills to be successful in public school. Additionally, district-supported interpreter services enabled students who used sign communication to be educated in mainstream environments as well. Mainstreaming for deaf children, as it is currently practiced, suggests that a child has sufficient language, literacy, and academic achievement to access the regular grade-level curriculum, with only minimal adaptations to the content, with or without support. Thus, a second grader placed in a classroom with a regular education teacher (with no training in deafness) and an educational interpreter is considered *mainstreamed.* The student will be expected to complete all assignments in the regular curriculum under the classroom teacher's direction and may receive only scheduled visits from an itinerant (traveling) teacher of deaf children.

The Relationship of Communication Choice and Placement Options

One might assume that it is relatively easy for parents to find an educational program that supports their communication choice. Unfortunately, there is not a one-to-one correspondence between communication choice and placement option. Not every placement is able to support any and all of the various communication methodologies that can be used by a child with hearing loss. For example, parents may choose to learn and use Cued Speech in the home but find there is no regional preschool program in place to receive their child after Early Intervention eligibility expires. Other parents may want their child to be placed in a Simultaneous Communication environment but find that the local day class program has adopted an oral/aural communication philosophy. It is here that the challenge of securing services for a child with a hearing loss is most clearly evident. Parents may be asked to acquiesce to the model of delivery that is common practice in the district. It is not unusual for the issue of communication to be the basis for litigation by parents who seek to change the status quo within a local board of education. Many parents of children with cochlear implants have faced similar difficulties in securing the proper combination of educational placement and communication option.

Educational Choices for Deaf Children with Implants

Some parents choose a cochlear implant as a tool for achieving the end goal of mainstream placement for their child. There is, in fact, literature to support the educational effectiveness of the implant in children. Published reports indicate that implantation reduces special education costs over time because children with implants can be mainstreamed earlier. This report, in effect, sets mainstreaming as the educational end goal in and of itself. Perhaps, however, it may be more prudent to view the end goal as what lies beyond mainstreaming: grade-level, linguistic, academic, and social competence. With this new target in mind, mainstreaming may not be the appropriate placement for every child. Therefore, mainstream placement should be viewed as only one of the *means* to an end. Other placement options exist that might be more appropriate than mainstreaming in helping children achieve their fullest potential. Let's explore each of the placement options and consider its appropriateness for a child with an implant.

Schools for Deaf Children

Schools for deaf children espouse different language and educational philosophies, so parents should become familiar with the special features of a particular program before they make their placement decision. The identifying characteristics of each placement type are outlined below.

State Schools for Deaf Children Using American Sign Language

The United States has a rich history of service delivery to students with hearing loss. After the opening of what is now the American School for the Deaf in 1817, states across the country systematically established residential schools in a central location to educate students with hearing loss. Although these schools may still have residential programs, large numbers of deaf children attend their state school as day students. It is at the state school that one will generally find the largest number of teachers and support personnel who are deaf. For this and other philosophical and instructional reasons, these schools have made a commitment to use American Sign Language (ASL) and an orientation to the development of Deaf culture, identity, and heritage in their students. Thus, the state school for deaf children will be a place where exposure to deaf role models can occur and where immersion in an environment that sees deafness as a difference and not a disability can take place. According to some researchers, students at residential schools for the deaf have better self-esteem and social sense of self than do students in mainstreamed environments. It is often argued that when a student attends a deaf school, leadership roles are more attainable because the deafness itself is not a barrier to be overcome. These schools are a community of individuals bound together by the linguistic and social world of deafness.

Until recently, students with implants in this type of setting had limited opportunity to use the device because the visual environment precluded the need for speaking and listening. These students wore their implants only during interactions with family and friends outside of school. State schools are now beginning to explore ways in which to deliver instruction to deaf students who use implants. Time will determine whether schools that have made an instructional commitment to ASL can philosophically support the implant with their current practices.

State residential schools may wish to act as resources to the large number of deaf students in other educational settings who are using implants to learn spoken English. As these students mature, they may seek to learn ASL and more about deafness and Deaf culture. No place is better equipped than the state residential school for reaching out to this community of implant recipients to impart the language and heritage of deaf individuals. It is hoped that schools for the deaf will assume this unique role in providing children with implants the link to deaf history.

Private Oral Schools for Deaf Children

A small number of private oral schools exists that provide education to day, and sometimes residential, students. These schools have historically taught deaf children by using the residual hearing available to them through their hearing aids. Strategies and techniques used at the schools in the past, when introduced to children using implants, appear appropriate and highly effective for learning spoken language. Sometimes, children who are implanted before three years of age will be enrolled in one of these private oral schools for intensive development of spoken language in the preschool years. If the program extends into the elementary grades, these children may continue to attend the primary years to firmly establish early reading skills. A given child's performance will dictate whether continued oral school placement, or placement in an included or mainstream setting, will lead to maximal educational achievement. Children who require individual or small group instruction that emphasizes particular oral communication strategies may make better academic progress in a classroom setting uniquely designed to accommodate their special auditory learning needs.

Day Schools for Deaf Children
Using Simultaneous Communication

In day schools that use the Simultaneous Communication method, children are exposed to spoken English that is supplemented by manual signs in English word order. Care must be taken when choosing schools that espouse this communication orientation. Because it is difficult to speak and sign at the same time, the quality of language input is sometimes compromised. In some circumstances, the child is neither seeing a complete representation of English on the hands nor hearing a complete spoken message from the mouth. It is wise to speak with the administrator of the Simultaneous Communication program to learn more about the implementation of the communication policy. Likewise, it may be helpful to observe the activities of the classroom to determine how this methodology is being practiced.

Schools that successfully implement this form of communication and have made a commitment to aggressive auditory management of the child with an implant are ideal placements for children to achieve their goals of academic and social success. In this type of educational setting, there is often a critical mass of students, so that small and homogeneous instructional groups contribute to a rigorous scholastic environment for those capable of meeting this challenge. Thus, it is not only in the mainstream that deaf students can have access to advanced coursework. Strategies and techniques that support learning for children with hearing loss are implemented directly by the class-room teacher rather than by interpreted or supported instruction in the mainstream. An additional advantage is that the students are exposed to important social issues related to deaf role models, cultural identity, and heritage because they are in a school for the deaf.

Regional Programs

In some circumstances, regional programs provide children with implants the widest array of choices within a single system. Unlike schools for deaf children that generally have a unified communication policy, some regional programs have both oral and sign tracks, and they offer a continuum of classroom settings from self-contained education to mainstream placement. In this model, the child with an implant may continue the communication program begun in Early Intervention and move within the placement options available in the system as opposed to moving between service delivery systems. For example, one regional program under the direction of a central administration may be able to provide small group instruction, including classroom placements, within-district mainstreaming, and itinerant support to a child mainstreamed out of district. These choices may be available in oral, simultaneous communication, and Cued Speech tracks.

Self-Contained Classes within a Public School
for Children with Implants

Districts offering day class services within a self-contained classroom to children with hearing loss are most vulnerable to the rise and fall of enrollment from year to year. This occurs because children move, age out of the program, or enter more mainstream-type settings. In addition, the communication philosophy may be rigid, since relatively small numbers of deaf children preclude the availability of an array of communication choices. For parents who are determined to have their children educated close to home, this format may be more appealing than the state school for the deaf. Self-contained placement may be more academically appropriate than inclusion, especially when the receiving classroom is beyond the linguistic and academic reach of a child.

Characteristics of Schools that Support Children with Implants

Regardless of the type of program in which a child is enrolled, a focus on speaking and listening on a daily basis is required to meet the needs of the child with an implant. In a supportive school environment, audition is valued as much for communication as it is as a tool for learning academics. Administrators have introduced professional development seminars to show their support for working with children with implants. Teachers and auxiliary personnel are knowledgeable of auditory skill development and make a commitment to integrate opportunities for listening and speaking into everyday classroom routines. This is established practice for children in auditory/oral environments, whether they are residential or day programs.

Children with implants in schools and programs that use Simultaneous Communication will need special attention throughout the school day. In order to maximize the use of the implant, some instruction must be delivered to the child in an auditory-only manner. This dictates that the teacher will consciously refrain from signing at certain times in order to provide the child with a genuine listening opportunity. Teachers attend professional development workshops to increase their knowledge and skills for incorporating listening opportunities into the classroom. Sometimes teachers are resistant to these oral-only activities out of concern for other children in the classroom who rely on sign for communication purposes. However, it is not sufficient for a child with an implant to practice listening in a pullout session with the speech pathologist. Experience suggests that the best results in developing listening skills and spoken language abilities are attained when students have ample opportunities to learn *through* listening rather than simply learning *to* listen.

Children with implants who attend state schools for the deaf present a unique challenge. Administrators of these programs have sought to focus on the role of ASL in reading and curriculum development. This commitment has effectively precluded them from actively participating in the education of deaf children with cochlear implants. In an attempt to maintain a competitive presence in the education of deaf children, more schools for the deaf are beginning to integrate children with implants by reconfiguring the activities of their early intervention and preschool programs to include more speaking and listening opportunities. It will take a generation of teachers and administrators to identify a place where the worlds of implantation and the state schools for the deaf can effectively meet.

Trends in the education of all children are evolving. More classrooms are using computer technology and audio-visual formats. Distance learning and computer chat rooms now provide children with access to information about a variety of subjects from teachers and places outside their immediate classroom walls. Models that encourage students to construct knowledge as a community of learners have replaced the traditional didactic method of presenting information. The classrooms of the future will look substantially different than those we know today. Advances in cochlear implant technology will likely outpace the changes in our classrooms thereby creating the potential for new and exciting ways to configure education for deaf children.

Chapter 9

Cochlear Implants and the Whole Child:
Implications for Performance

hildren with cochlear implants demonstrate abilities that often astound parents, teachers, and the children themselves. But not every child with an implant performs in the same manner. What may be success for one child might be viewed as failure for another. Parents should understand that their child's performance with the implant is often linked to the skills and abilities the child had when he or she entered the implant process. The more children *bring* to the process, the more they will *gain* from it.

Generally speaking, children with implants demonstrate a range of performance in speech perception and speech production. Auditorily, children with implants can be grouped into three main categories. At the extreme low end are those children who can only detect or recognize sound patterns. For these children, implantation only provides an awareness of sound; they cannot understand spoken language through listening alone. The next level of performance includes children who are able to understand some speech through their implants but still need visual or manual cues to participate in conversations. The highest performing group is made up of those children who can understand speech through listening alone. Despite this good auditory success, these children may still need speechreading cues to comprehend speech, especially in noise.

Just how intelligible a child's speech becomes after implantation also varies. At the extreme low end, there is a group of children whose speech will remain unintelligible. This is followed by a group of children whose speech is understandable as long as the listener knows the topic of the conversation. Finally, there is a group of implant users whose speech is completely understandable, even to strangers. More often than not, it is likely that a child's speaking success is related to listening ability.

In the chapter that discussed the pre-implant evaluation, we identified a number of factors that shape performance. These were outlined using the tool known as the ChIP (see chapter 2). Beyond the factors identified by the ChIP are additional issues that contribute to any one child's implant benefit. To begin with, parents should remember that no two children, whether hearing or deaf, are the same. Each one brings a personality, level of motivation, and general outlook about the world to the process. These traits affect how a child approaches every experience and can also influence the auditory gains achieved after implantation. Videotapes distributed by manufacturers or organizations and schools that champion implantation often show children who are the better performers. Parents considering the implant cannot use these films as the only resource to make predictions about their own child's performance. This may lead to disappointment for everyone involved. *The numerous factors that affect implant performance make it virtually impossible to determine the exact outcome any particular child will achieve.* Thus, it is important for parents to understand implant performance considering the "whole child" and not just the "ears."

Factors Contributing to Implant Performance

As we noted in the discussion on candidacy, age at the time of implantation and duration of deafness are two critical factors that can affect performance with an implant. When children receive an implant after a short duration of deafness, then achievement tends to reach the high end of the scale. This does not mean that children with a longer duration of deafness cannot receive implants. It just means that the results may not be as great or achieved as quickly as a child who had a shorter duration of deafness. It is obvious that children who are implanted earlier in life will, by definition, have a shorter duration of deafness. Recall, the U.S. Food and Drug Administration has approved implantation in profoundly deaf children as early as twelve months of age. Some children have received implants in infancy due to special medical circumstances (e.g., severe cochlear ossification secondary to early meningitis), thereby exploring the potential for even earlier implantation. The implantation of this younger group is recent and, therefore, analysis of follow-up data is not yet possible. Preliminary results indicate that these deaf infants develop auditory skills in a manner that is more similar to hearing children their own age. The ultimate effect this will have on the development of speech and language skills is being studied at the present time and shows great promise.

As the age of the congenitally (from birth) deaf child increases, the duration of deafness increases. This is also true for the prelinguistically deafened (before the development of language, usually before two years of age) child. Depending upon the duration of deafness, there may be a substantial delay in the development of many listening and speaking skills. Supporters of the use of American Sign Language (ASL) insist that deaf children refrain from receiving implants until they are older. This may seriously reduce the benefits of implantation, especially for children beyond the language-learning years. In other words, children who are implanted later in life will not be able to demonstrate considerable improvements in their spoken language skills. They may, however, receive benefit through changes in auditory awareness. In some cases, this may be a sufficient goal for parents or child. In other cases, it may not.

In addition to the age at implantation and the duration of deafness, there are other factors that affect implant performance.

These factors are explained below.

Factors That Affect Implant Performance Outcomes Beyond Age at Implantation and Duration of Deafness

- structure of the cochlea,
- presence of disabilities,
- presence and sophistication of a formal language system,
- expectations of the parents and the child,
- amount and quality of family support,
- educational environment,
- availability and quality of support services,
- wear-time of the device,
- duration of implant use,
- presence of a second language in the home,
- proper functioning of the device, and
- appropriate adjustment of the device.

Structure of the Cochlea

Children who have cochleae with significant bone growth (ossification) after meningitis are capable of obtaining good benefit from the use a cochlear implant. However, if the amount of cochlear ossification is so great that very little of the signal reaches the auditory nerve, the benefit that the child receives may be limited. Also, some children may not reach adequate performance levels if the meningitis affected physical or cognitive functioning.

Children with malformed cochleae may also demonstrate good performance. In some cases, however, the degree of malformation affects the auditory nerve, resulting in poorer performance. This group of children often exhibits a higher occurrence of facial nerve stimulation (involuntary facial movement with auditory stimulation). Facial nerve stimulation may be resolved by eliminating electrodes or reducing power to them; but this may limit the implant's performance since adequate electrode stimulation is not possible.

It is reassuring to know that, like children with ossification, children who do not have perfectly formed cochleae are capable of receiving implants and obtaining benefit. Parents need to keep in mind, though, that these structural differences may prevent their child from achieving high performance with the implant.

Presence of Disabilities

A variety of physical and cognitive disabilities, ranging from the presence of low muscle tone to developmental disabilities, can affect a child's success with an implant. The extent of the disability will have an impact on the degree of benefit that a child may obtain with an implant. Disabilities that are noncognitive in nature, for example blindness, may have no effect on ultimate auditory benefit. Those disabilities that are cognitive in nature may make the use of an implant inappropriate.

Children with cognitive disabilities such as pervasive developmental delay, mental retardation, and autism may receive only minimal benefit from a cochlear implant and, in some cases, no benefit at all. Experiences with these children have been limited since implantation was initially reserved for children without disabilities. Research indicates that, if implanted early, some children with milder degrees of cognitive involvement may demonstrate better attention, respond to surrounding sounds more consistently, and be more connected with their environment. Under no circumstances, have these children developed the speaking and listening skills similar to the larger implant population. Parents of children with cognitive disabilities often report that addressing the hearing loss through implantation allowed them to focus on the child's cognitive needs at an earlier stage of development.

Children with noncognitive disabilities such as blindness, mild forms of cerebral palsy, or low muscle tone have made substantial progress with their implants, especially when implanted at a young age. The presence of learning disabilities and attention deficit disorders will affect performance much in the same manner that they do in the hearing population. Once again, parents of children with any of these issues should discuss them carefully and openly during the pre-implant period. As parents seek implantation for their deaf infants, they must be alerted to the fact that their children may, at later ages, exhibit disabilities unrelated to deafness. It is almost impossible to detect problems such as attention deficit disorder or learning disabilities in young babies. These may or may not have an effect on the performance of children with an implant. Implantation may, however, assist parents in obtaining treatment for the learning challenge in a more timely fashion instead of attributing the behavior to deafness.

Presence and Sophistication of a Formal Language System

Cochlear implants perform best when the chronological age and the language age (age equivalent assigned to the child's language performance) of the recipient are closely matched. This is the main reason that so many postlinguistically deafened adults and children have enjoyed such success with implants. Conversely, children with large differences in chronological and linguistic age will do poorer than expected. It is critically important for children to have a formal language system and to perform at a level that is within sight of their hearing agemates. When a gap between chronological and language age occurs (which is typical of deaf children) it should be no more than a few years in duration. Language competence can be demonstrated either orally and/or through manual codes of English. In fact, many parents begin using sign language with their children to ensure that they have access to vocabulary and syntax at an early age.

These children often continue to use their signing skills after implantation to accrue new knowledge and to support their listening and speaking skills.

Competence in ASL must be viewed relative to the age at implantation and the duration of deafness. Congenitally deaf adolescents who use ASL as their only form of communication will not likely understand the acoustic information provided through the implant to its fullest. This occurs because the auditory input is English and the sign input is ASL. Young children who present with emerging ASL abilities may be considered for implantation as long as there is a commitment to use spoken English to develop their listening skills.

Expectations of the Parents and the Child

All parents expect their children to perform better with an implant than with their hearing aids. If they did not hold this belief, the decision to implant would not have been made in the first place. Parents have reported that their level of expectation changes throughout the process. Some expectations change in a positive direction while others change in a negative direction. Parents and children who approach implantation with unrealistic goals will find the early days of implant use filled with much discouragement. This is especially true for adolescents. It is not unusual for teenagers to view implantation as a path toward more intelligible speech. Although this is a worthy goal, it is not one that can be reached early in the process. For many teenagers who receive an implant, significant speech changes occur only after years of implant use. If the adolescent recipient is not prepared for this delayed gratification, he or she runs the risk of disappointment and eventual nonuse. Even when expectations are appropriate, there will be intervals during which no new auditory or speech abilities will develop. This "slump" is usually temporary and requires that both parent and child work through these periods with a positive attitude.

Parents of very young implant recipients sometimes notice a similar plateau as the child's language and speech skills struggle to reach the level of their auditory abilities. As long as parents continue to support their children with maximal auditory and spoken language input, these plateaus will be overcome. Persistent problems, however, should be investigated to ensure that there is not another cause for the setback, such as equipment malfunction. One thing is clear: regardless of the age of the implant user, if the parent or child believes that the implant no longer provides benefit, then, in all likelihood, it will not. This "self-fulfilling prophecy" can seriously affect performance and must be guarded against.

Amount and Quality of Family Support

The support of family sustains children through the entire process—from candidacy through long-term use. The role that parents play can never be overemphasized. It is the parents who reinforce listening and speaking activities learned at school. It is the parents who help the child through the periods of "performance plateaus" that occur. But parents need not be alone in their support of the child with the implant. The entire extended family can be asked to encourage the child's successful use of the implant. The role that siblings, grandparent, aunts, and uncles play can further enrich the listening experiences of the child to reinforce implant use. Families that understand how the implant works will challenge the child to listen and speak without being too demanding or too easy.

Families that do not take the time to enhance the implant user's spoken language and listening skills, place the child at risk for diminished performance. In some circumstances, families are unable to effectively provide the child with the needed stimulation because of parents' schedules or siblings' needs. In other cases, families believe that it is the school's responsibility to provide all the stimulation that is required for implant benefit. Regardless of the reason for the lack of home support, the child loses out on valuable experiences that can assist in developing better skills.

Conversely, those families that continually require the child to respond with an auditory or spoken behavior are fulfilling two needs. The first is the exposure to oral language that will add to the child's experience. The second, and more important need, is integrating the child into the family by making him or her a natural part of conversations that take place. Children who come from supportive households are exposed to more opportunities to use their skills and to sharpen them over time.

Educational Environment

In chapter 8, the emphasis on the role of the educational environment was discussed at great length. It is important for parents to understand the power the educational setting has on their child's performance with an implant. For example, parents who wish their children to develop spoken language skills as their primary communication mode may be more inclined to enroll their children in programs with an auditory/oral orientation. Other parents may have a broader focus and choose the implant as an overall communication tool that complements a simultaneous communication environment. Parents must remember that the school's primary goal is to teach their children content material. In some cases, this can be accomplished using an oral-only approach. In other cases, sign language may be used in conjunction with spoken language to teach subject matter. Children with cochlear implants can thrive in either environment; gaining maximum benefit from the device requires that the child be continually challenged to use listening and speaking skills as often as possible. Up to this point in time, schools for deaf children that use only ASL have provided rich academic environments but have been unable to effectively challenge the listening and speaking skills of children with implants. In fact, children who received implants in the mid- to late-1980s and were enrolled in these programs often became nonusers.

Parents must remember that no one type of educational setting fits every child. Some children will require a multisensory approach to maximize both their learning potential and their implant use. Other children may perform well with a unisensory (auditory-only) approach. What is important is that parents understand that their child's ultimate performance with a cochlear implant will be the result of an accumulation of auditory experiences that occur throughout the day. When there is less exposure, there is less opportunity for children with implants to use their skills. Less opportunity often means less benefit.

Availability and Quality of Support Services

Although some professionals lead parents to believe that only one type of therapy creates success with a cochlear implant, children have benefited using any one of a variety of methodologies. As more children are implanted and parents become knowledgeable about the needs of their children, school districts are scrambling to identify appropriate professionals to provide services. Although the number of professionals with *knowledge* in the field of implantation has grown, there may still be only a limited number of speech/language pathologists, audiologists, or teachers of deaf children who have *experience* working with implanted children. A good alternative, however, is to identify a professional who is skilled in providing services to children with hearing loss. Generally, these are speech/language pathologists who have worked with children using traditional amplification. Therapy with cochlear implants is similar to the more traditional auditory, speech, and language work that speech/language pathologists are accustomed to performing with many hard of hearing children. Therapists who have worked with children who were profoundly deaf and used hearing aids often note the most significant change is the relative ease with which the child with an implant acquires auditory and speech skills. This new capacity prompts the professional to stimulate the child implant user to strive for greater auditory, speech, and language proficiency earlier in the process of habilitation.

Wear-Time of the Device

Performance with a cochlear implant improves with use of the device over time. It becomes critical, therefore, that children utilize the implant for as many waking hours as possible. Children whose wear-time is limited only to school hours are decreasing their amount of exposure to sound, which ultimately restricts performance. When children do not consistently use their implants at home, families lose valuable time and experience that can reinforce listening. Since the sounds at home are so crucial to everyday activity, this missed opportunity will affect overall benefit. Children with implants require constant auditory and spoken language input. The only way this can be accomplished is by consistent use of the device.

Children, especially adolescents, who begin to reduce wear-time run the risk of becoming nonusers. For this reason, parents of teenagers should be diligent in monitoring their child's implant use. The improved cosmetics of the external speech processor—from a body-worn device to one that is smaller and sits behind the ear like a traditional hearing aid—has made wear-time less of an issue for this population. Regardless of the age of the implant user or the outward appearance of the speech processor, the more time a child wears the cochlear implant, the greater the benefit.

Duration of Implant Use

Related to the wear-time of the device is the concept of duration of implant use. As children wear implants over time, performance will improve. Parents report that even after years of implantation, their child will acknowledge the detection of new sounds. Parents at the beginning of the habilitative process are often eager to see marked changes in behaviors. This does not always occur and may cause dismay when one child does not demonstrate the same amount of progress that another child shows during a similar time period. It is important for parents to remember that each child, whether hearing or deaf, progresses at his or her own pace. It is equally important for parents to understand that as duration of implant use increases so does implant benefit. The rate of progress may vary substantially from child to child, with each child reaching maximum performance levels at different times as a result of individual differences.

Presence of a Second Language in the Home

It is not unusual for a percentage of children who receive implants to come from home environments in which a second language is spoken. Some families of implanted children may not speak any English, may have limited command of English, or may be fluent in English and another language. Children who are schooled in English-speaking academic environments during the day and return home to another language may demonstrate some delay in the acquisition of each language. In many cases, especially for children implanted early, there will be a certain degree of proficiency in both languages. Children often develop two sets of vocabulary; one set to reflect the language of the home and the other to reflect the language of the classroom. This is common for children who learn English as a second language.

Children who return to a household in which English and another language are spoken will also develop skills in both languages and will also demonstrate a delay in one or both languages. More research is necessary in this area to determine the depth of proficiency that children acquire in each of the languages and whether a dominant language can be identified. Implant teams and/or schools may differ substantially in their philosophy towards the presence of a second language at home. Some might suggest that only English be spoken while others will reinforce the development of the two languages with the full knowledge that a delay may occur. Clearly, as more children receive implants from multilingual homes, there will be more data to support or refute some of these recommendations.

Proper Functioning of the Device

A cochlear implant can only benefit a child if the device is functioning within specifications. Implants that are intermittently or poorly maintained do not deliver a consistent signal; consequently, the implant's effectiveness is reduced. If parents, teachers, therapists, and children do not monitor the function of the equipment every day, poor performance may result. Implants should be checked daily for problems related to the cords, microphone, and battery power to ensure that the best signal is being delivered. These types of checks should be a routine part of the child's home, academic, and therapeutic life.

Appropriate Adjustment of the Device

In addition to functioning properly, a cochlear implant must also be tuned correctly. Children whose implants are poorly tuned will not demonstrate the same performance gains as children whose devices are properly tuned. It is important that children be remapped at the periodic intervals recommended by the implant facility. Children who are incorrectly mapped will not have the best access to the speech signal. Without that access, children will be unable to make the finer discriminations that are necessary to develop the auditory and spoken language skills that are possible with the implant. Even in cases in which the child lives a distance from the implant center, parents must make a commitment to return regularly to ensure that the device is properly set. If this is not done, the child will not reach his or her fullest potential. When children are local to the implant facility, any change in performance can be reported and resolved quickly.

What Is Implant "Success"?

The entire issue of implantation is integrally linked to performance. Supporters of implantation point to the good outcomes demonstrated by implant users; opponents of implantation can find numerous examples of implant "failures." This begs the question, "Must *everyone* be a better-than-average performer in order to preserve implantation as a viable option for *anyone*?" The very notion of demanding that more children perform in the "better-than-average" category defies the definition of "average." Further, as noted previously, there are several mitigating circumstances that affect the benefit an implant affords any child.

First and foremost, it is important to remember what an implant can and cannot do. It may be helpful to think of the implant as a sound messenger. This sound messenger delivers auditory signals to the central processing headquarters of the brain. For children with implants, this is the best that can be expected—that sound will get to the brain. The work of the implant is finished at that time, and then the messenger awaits another message. Once in the brain, the delivered sound or message is interpreted and acted upon. An implant has no effect at this central level. Thus, deaf children who use implants and also demonstrate cognitive deficits or other language-processing disorders will have the same problems faced by hearing children with these issues. Sound gets in, but doesn't get used in the same manner as by the cognitively intact child or the child with normal language ability.

A functioning cochlear implant, delivering signals to an intact central processing system, should enable a child to demonstrate auditory ability somewhere on the continuum of possible auditory outcomes. More importantly, a child will often outperform him- or herself, demonstrating greater auditory skills than would have been possible with traditional hearing aids. Exactly where any one child will place on the continuum will more likely be the result of factors outlined above rather than the auditory potential of the implant. It makes sense that any group of children, implant users or not, will be affected by learning challenges and home environment issues.

What Is Implant "Failure"?

The term *implant failure* has been used in a number of different contexts; parents who are considering implantation for their child should be fully informed with regard to this term. In its most literal sense, the internal components of the implant may fail and the device will cease to perform properly. When this occurs, the most frequent course of action is another surgery. Others have used the term *implant failure* to refer to situations in which a child rejects the device and no longer uses it. These are youngsters who, for some reason, choose not to wear the implant. Issues that may cause a child to cease wearing the implant can be categorized as cosmetic, environmental, or related to poorer-than-expected performance outcomes.

Because it was believed that young adults or teenagers would best mirror the success of the adult population of implant users, they were among the first pediatric recipients. The actual experience with these adolescents was rather disappointing as a myriad of issues combined to create a negative attitude about implant use. The cosmetics of the early implant device, a large body-worn processor, interfered with its acceptance and use. Educational environments that did not unconditionally accept a child with an implant sent a not-so-subtle message about the value of the device and the child wearing it. In an effort to "fit in," implant recipients would decrease wear-time, until the self-fulfilling prophecy of receiving little or no benefit came to fruition. This type of *implant failure* was perhaps emotional, not mechanical; when there was little to listen to, there was no point in wearing an auditory device.

In some cases, parents did not include their teenager in the decision-making process, so teenagers found themselves implanted without a voice in the matter. Often, shortly after implantation, these individuals purposely and actively removed external equipment to demonstrate their philosophical stance on implant technology. A final group of implant users, who approached implantation with unusually high expectations, ceased using the device due to limited benefit. While it is more than likely that some cause could be found for the limited benefit, identifying a specific reason for any one individual is probably irrelevant. At the point in time at which the decision to stop using an implant occurs, there is no way to motivate a user to keep trying.

Young children are not likely to challenge implant use in the wake of limited benefit. Experience suggests that adolescent users who receive minimal benefit most often stop wearing the device. It is important to realize that individual choice and dissatisfaction with the device may lead an implant recipient to discontinue using it. It is always an option not to wear the external equipment. Can this be called implant "failure?"

When parents make decisions for their child, at any age, they believe they are acting in the child's best interests. When they choose implants, parents should know that children who receive sufficient benefit from the device will be motivated to continue wearing it. They should also be aware of the fact that children receiving limited benefit from the device will be unmotivated to use it. There is no way that parents or professionals can determine the level of performance that must be achieved to motivate the child. The level of performance that one child finds motivating may not be sufficient for another child.

Parents who choose an implant for their child would be well advised to put the implant in a larger perspective and consider it a tool, not a "miracle." Many life experiences will contribute to the person the child will ultimately become. Parents should keep their "eyes on the prize" of raising a child with good self-esteem, who achieves his or her full potential, whatever that may be, and feels the love and acceptance of a nurturing family.

Chapter 10

Deaf Culture and the Cochlear Implant

The cochlear implant has changed the way the medical community looks at deafness. While historically seen as a condition that could only be marginally treated, deafness is now approached with a more optimistic prognosis. The cochlear implant has revolutionized treatment for thousands of children and adults with profound hearing loss. This technology, however, has not been embraced by the Deaf community, who sees no reason to "treat" deafness. This comes as no surprise since previous "treatments," such as hearing aids, were also rejected. This tension between the Deaf and medical communities has resurfaced as the implant has gained popular acceptance.

It is natural to have conflict within any society. This dissension may be attributed to religious, cultural, political, or personal life experiences. There are numerous ways an individual can cope with differences between and among groups in society. On one end of the continuum are those who are unaware of any controversy and therefore have no opinion and take no action. On the opposite end are those who are unshakeable in their beliefs and resistant to any change. These individuals may, in fact, hold so strongly to their belief system that they take radical action against those holding a different viewpoint. They are often vocal, interpret facts in a narrow manner that supports their beliefs, and work actively to convince others to join their crusade. Between these two endpoints is the larger population of individuals who are determined to arrive at an informed position and struggle to wade through the rhetoric of the extremists to arrive at a balanced viewpoint.

It is unlikely that persons who are either indifferent or highly passionate about a particular issue or belief can be easily swayed toward middle ground. Groups that occupy points within the continuum have a greater chance of developing an appreciation and respect for different views. Movement along the continuum can occur in either direction as new facts are uncovered and new experiences are gained. In order to embrace alternative positions, individuals must be open to adding new information to their knowledge base. Developing an informed position is the result of information gathering from a variety of independent sources and taking an objective look at the facts.

Deafness and the positions on deafness held by hearing and deaf people can also be drawn along a continuum. On one end are hearing people who know and care little about deafness because it does not directly affect their lives. On the other end are deaf activists who are passionate about their deafness and regard any attempt to change the audiological circumstance of deafness as unnecessary. Furthermore, treating deafness as a medical condition and not a cultural difference is considered an assault on the Deaf community. Not surprisingly, it is this core group of the Deaf community that has served as the catalyst for bringing the linguistic, social, and political issues of deafness to the forefront of society at large. The current generation of deaf individuals has seen American Sign Language (ASL) achieve stature as a legitimate language. High schools and colleges across the United States offer ASL among their courses to meet world language requirements.

Other forces have shaped the experiences of the Deaf community today. Most deaf individuals recall where they were in 1988, when the Deaf President Now (DPN) movement erupted on the Gallaudet University campus. This event brought national and international attention to the issues of the Deaf community. For the first time, many individuals in the United States took notice of deaf people and their cause. The controversy centered on the appointment of a hearing person to the position of president of the university. The subsequent appointment of I. King Jordan as the first deaf president of this institution was a hard-won victory for the community. From this event, recognition of the Deaf community as a viable political and social force evolved. As a constituency, they are now counted as a political base to be courted. Equal access to government and political activities is ensured through the availability of sign language interpreters at major events. Socially, deaf persons can access many more activities because of the accommodations mandated by the Americans with Disabilities Act (ADA). Theatrical performances and movies can be enjoyed through sign interpreting or captioning. Movies, television dramas, and even soap operas have story lines that involve deaf issues and star deaf actors or actresses. All new televisions have built-in decoders, and the majority of shows are captioned. Many hearing individuals have appreciated the presence of this technology to assist in their television viewing. These achievements have come through the hard work of the Deaf community activists who have committed time and energy to the advancement of deaf causes.

The personal histories of these individuals are rich in the traditions of deafness, and their accomplishments in society are numerous and diverse. These men and women are often the children, grandchildren, and great-grandchildren of deaf parents, deaf grandparents and deaf great-grandparents, creating a tradition of deafness with a worldview from a deaf perspective. Their lives have been normalized with deafness as the referent. While many positive changes to the deaf experience have been accomplished by technology, the debut of the cochlear implant on the heels of the DPN movement interrupted the savoring of the victory won on the Gallaudet campus. These opposing forces emerging at the same time laid the foundation for the new "cold war" between hearing and deaf individuals.

Given the worldview of deaf activists, cochlear implants are rejected because they pose a threat to the deaf experience. In fact, members of the Deaf community rightfully resent a hearing worldview that cannot appreciate their personal opposition to the technology. Naïve members of the hearing community expect that implants would be welcomed by all persons who are deaf. Documentaries such as *Sound and Fury* have begun to educate hearing people about the perspective that the Deaf community holds relative to cochlear implant technology. But this is a two-way street. Staunch deaf activists cannot appreciate hearing parents whose own tradition of hearing causes them to seek implantation for their deaf child. Some members of the Deaf community attem⸻

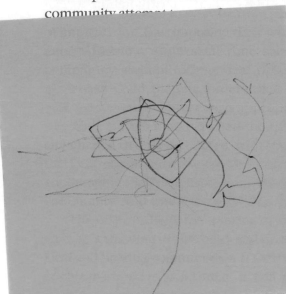

rents away from the choice rldview on the hearing par- e members of the hearing ts of deaf children to im- hearing worldview on the ate nor effective and leads groups. This jeopardizes lants will be accepted by ide hearing parents from lants to explore the Deaf drawn.

tunities for and not *bar-* be shared equally by the mmunity members view vent them from taking ⸻those children who receive them. Similarly, hearing parents should recognize that Deaf community members are able to provide their deaf child with something they cannot, and that is experience as a deaf person. Up to now, the Deaf community's position has used cases of implant failure as the reason to withhold implantation from all children. The hearing community's position seizes upon every implant success to validate a recommendation to provide the implant to all children. Each community must recognize the range of performance that can be achieved after implantation and appreciate the fact that, in some cases, each position is the correct one.

At the current time, deaf individuals with hearing aids or implants whose lack of spoken language abilities preclude them from taking an active place in the hearing community often turn to the Deaf community for identity. This reinforces the Deaf community's view that amplification and implantation are unsuccessful. High performing implanted children whose spoken language abilities are well developed become fully integrated into the hearing community, thus preventing their exploration of deafness-related issues. The hearing community's view of implantation as a necessary tool for deaf children is reinforced while, at the same time, the role of the Deaf community in raising a "whole" deaf child is overlooked.

While it may be presumptuous for those in the field of implantation to call upon the Deaf community to reach out to deaf children with implants, it is our intent to do just that. Although the process of cochlear implantation may still be considered deplorable by many, the National Association of the Deaf's second position paper represents a shift from its earlier hard-line stance on implants in children. This may be, in part, a response to the trend that indicates that hearing parents are choosing implantation for their deaf children in growing numbers. While the motivation for this tendency may be multifaceted, the majority of youngsters with severe to profound deafness are receiving implants soon after they reach the age criterion. Early implantation provides these children with the potential to grow and learn with a "cochlear implant worldview" that is both hearing and deaf. Perhaps, it is this generation that may provide the bridge between the deaf and hearing worlds if each will allow it to happen. Energy spent in defending viewpoints and recruiting other supporters to one side of the controversy or the other may be better spent when channeled into consensus building between opponents and proponents of implantation for children. Borrowing from the political world, perhaps it is time for "bipartisan" efforts on behalf of children with implants so that opportunities are created "on both sides of the aisle" without diminishing the fundamental belief system of either group. This effort will only serve to benefit the very children we are fighting over—the next generation of deaf adults.

Just how can this new world order be accomplished? Since the implant has been the catalyst for returning deaf issues to the forefront, it is incumbent upon cochlear implant centers to make the effort to understand the deaf perspective. This should be mirrored by similar efforts on the part of Deaf community members. Putting these initiatives into action can take several forms, some of which are offered as a starting point for discussion here.

- Implant centers can begin by collaborating with Deaf community members to establish programs that highlight the accomplishments of deaf individuals. For example, the implant center can identify a cadre of deaf persons who periodically make presentations to children with implants and their families on topics related to deaf heritage.
- Deaf presenters should be open, genuine, and supportive of hearing parents who have chosen implantation for their child because it was the right thing to do for their family tradition; these sessions should convey positive information about Deaf culture, not negative attitudes about the choice that was already made by parents.
- Implant center staff should appreciate the fact that deaf individuals are not interested in implant technology and should not attempt to change their minds!
- Members of deaf clubs may hold special meetings at implant centers and invite families with implanted children to discuss issues relating to deafness and deaf heritage with voice interpreting available.
- Implant centers should team with Deaf community members to create a website that will attract children

with implants and their parents; these websites can provide links to other established deaf-related websites.

- Implant centers can encourage deaf children with implants, their hearing siblings, and their parents to learn ASL as a second language and provide the resources to support such classes.
- Joint efforts between implant centers and the Deaf community could result in learning weekends that include children with and without implants.
- Implant centers can create a lending library stocked with books written by deaf authors describing their experiences.
- Implant centers may collaborate with schools for deaf children and sponsor social gatherings for all deaf children in the area.

It may be possible to envision a world in which all prejudices disappear and the inclination to dissent with others different from us diminishes. In this world, choices that individuals make are respected; agreements to disagree replace pressure to conform to a solitary view. While this world may be a lifetime away for the majority of those who read this book, it may be possible within the lifetime of our own children for whom we now make decisions. Perhaps all our deaf children will someday read this book and wonder what the controversy was about as they move freely within and/or between the deaf and hearing worlds. As parents of these deaf children, it is important to recognize that today's children are tomorrow's parents. The responsibility of raising tolerant and well-rounded individuals is not to be taken lightly.

Chapter 11

A Perspective on Parenting

The challenges that parents face everyday are magnified when a child has an identifiable difference. In some cases, this difference may be hearing loss. Although hearing parents of deaf children and hearing parents of hearing children confront many of the same issues, the presence of hearing loss will, for the most part, change the family dynamic from the moment it is detected. While books on parenting deaf children recommend that parents treat the child as a child first, parents are often unable to see beyond the deafness during the period immediately following identification. The immobilization that may occur after a child's hearing loss is identified can disrupt the natural course of bonding and communication between parent and child. Some parents, paralyzed by indecision, may feel pressure from professionals who urge them into action on behalf of their child. Time-sensitive issues such as obtaining hearing aids, learning a new method of communication, and enrolling the child in an early intervention program leave little room for delay. The responsibility to manage equipment, change accustomed communication practices, and take the baby to "school" are beyond the activities envisioned by parents when they were still parents-to-be. Inability to shoulder this unanticipated situation may make parents feel inadequate at best and guilt-ridden at worst as they struggle to meet a parenting challenge they never expected.

Parents who read this book are considering a cochlear implant for their child. Questions they have about implants are not answered in the popular parenting literature. As we undertook the task of writing this book, we decided to turn to the experts on parenting a child with a cochlear implant: the many wonderful families we have had the unique pleasure of meeting during our years at Lenox Hill Hospital and Manhattan Eye, Ear and Throat Hospital. The overwhelming response to our request made it obvious that there was much wisdom to be shared directly from the parents. Thus, with only minimal editing, we ask our parents to speak for themselves, as they answered many of the questions that have been included in this book.

Should We Choose Cochlear Implantation for Our Child?

This is probably one of the most difficult decisions we had to make concerning our daughter. My husband kept reminding me that the surgery was elective; it was not a life or death situation. But since I had already had the benefit of seeing many cochlear implant children and adult recipients, I kept emphasizing that it was a change in her "quality of life" as well as ours.

Research is key. Do your homework. Speak to parents of children with implants. Speak to people who have implants. Join organizations like AG Bell and CI Circle. Make the decision based on the FACTS: The greater the opportunities or tools given to your child, the more he is able to do with them. What he does with them is up to him when he is old enough to make decisions.

Cristina was diagnosed at four months of age as having a profound bilateral hearing loss. Although my husband's sister is also profoundly deaf, she can speak very well and learned how to speak Spanish and English in addition to her native Portuguese. So, our desire was that Cristina have the same opportunity to learn to speak and listen and to become independent. At six months of age, Cristina was fit with a body-worn hearing aid that did not seem to help her to recognize sounds despite my constant efforts to help her make the connection. . . . As time went on, Cristina continued not to show signs of detecting sounds even when using a powerful hearing aid coupled with an FM system. She was doing very well acquiring sign language, but very poorly in developing any awareness of sounds, or even understanding that she could produce sounds on her own. . . . She only detected sounds through vibrations. That took us to try a vibrotactile device called Tactaid . . . but the use of this device was limited to quiet environments. We had heard from the social worker at the center where she was initially diagnosed that [the] cochlear implant seemed to be a natural progression in our attempts to give her the tools to become more successful socially. . . . In the mean time, Cristina started to show more pronounced difficulties in seeing in the dark. . . . So as we went through the screening for the cochlear implant, we also got Cristina's diagnosis of Usher's Syndrome-Type 1 confirmed.

I knew the moment I was informed about the cochlear implant that it was my son's best hope for hearing my voice and the world around him.

We knew the implant was the way to go. We were just nervous about subjecting our eighteen-month-old to a two-and-a-half-hour surgery. We have never regretted the choice we made.

For us, there was no decision after weighing the risks vs. benefits. We whole-heartedly decided to go for whatever hearing that Matt could be offered by the implant.

At the time, it was an overwhelming decision because I was concerned about the long-term effects of the implant (i.e., device failure, etc.). Now, one-and-a-half years later, the implant has profoundly changed our daughter's quality of life, making me wonder why I even had a second thought.

That was just the next logical step for Spencer as hearing aids were not enough to help him acquire speech. Pursuing technology that is available is the next step when faced with an issue in the health care area.

Jeremy was a borderline case. We spent hours and hours talking to his therapists and audiologists. While he was receiving excellent benefit from an FM, he was behind in language. Children that we observed that were already implanted knew their colors, numbers, etc. Jeremy could only count to three, etc.

The day after our son was diagnosed, we learned of the implant from a newspaper article that my sister read. Thus, we always saw it as a possibility for our son and pursued it actively from the beginning. Nonetheless, we had concerns about the actual surgical procedure and wanted to be sure he really needed the implant before subjecting him to an invasive procedure.

As soon as we found out that our daughter was deaf, a cochlear implant was mentioned to us. We researched and knew it was what we wanted for her.

I was watching TV and saw a program talking about cochlear implants, so I called Lenox Hill to find out about it. I saw the Mets baseball player's child in the program.

When we originally found out our son was deaf, we hoped that we wouldn't have to make the decision about whether he would need an implant, as we hoped hearing aids alone would give him enough ability to hear. After it became obvious that hearing aids alone would not be enough to give him the capability for spoken language development, making the decision to get an implant for our son was actually quite easy to do. We had already made the decision that we wanted to give him every opportunity to develop spoken language capability in order to provide him with more opportunities in life. Given this goal, that left little choice but to go with the implant.... We still experienced tremendous anxiety over the actual CI surgery.

What Was the First Visit
to the Implant Center Like?

Once I convinced my husband to "explore the possibilities," we went to visit the local surgeon. I had already educated myself somewhat on the criteria for candidacy and asked various questions, listening to the surgeon's responses. Our local surgeon suggested we come back when our child was eight years old. This caused me to search for centers out of the area. A friend of mine provided us with the top ten eye and ear clinics and surgeons. We made appointments with the two closest facilities to us in New York City (a six-hour drive from our town). We had a list of questions that we asked both surgeons and personnel at the centers. Ultimately, it came down to whom we felt most comfortable with and who would support us in the long run.

First, we went to a different implant center from where we actually ended up. You are in such a fog at the beginning: You need medical advice—but from people who are sensitive to what you are going through. This is where you have to think about the ongoing support you will need and beyond just the surgery and device. Although difficult, this is the shortest phase of the process. The mapping and ongoing support is the longest and most important phase. Consequently, the people who will be working with you on an ongoing basis are of extreme importance.

Everyone at the center was friendly and helpful, and they followed Louie's progress closely. We went for three days of testing twice a year for six years after the original surgery. After the second implant surgery (after the first device failed), we try to go twice a year when Louie is home from college to check his mapping. The people at the new center have always been very nice and helpful if we asked for anything, but we are fairly self-sufficient and do not require much additional help.

Of course, I was very nervous about it. My husband stayed home with our older daughter, and we were going not only to have her evaluated for a cochlear implant but also to have her diagnosis of Usher's Syndrome confirmed. I was very worried that [because of] having a progressive visual disability on top of her profound hearing loss that her educational and professional possibilities would be narrowed. We stayed in New York for four days, and it all seemed to go too fast for me, but to proceed quickly [with the implant] seemed to make a lot of sense to me.

I really didn't know what to expect.

We were very anxious and hopeful that this would be the answer [for] our son. We watched other families and children and realized we were still numb from the realization we were now part of a new world.

We were trying not to get our hopes up that Matt would be a candidate for the implant.

The first visit was with the doctor. We would recommend that the audiologist and the team meet with the family first and then have the family meet with the doctor.

We felt like we were entering a "temple" for hearing disorders. We were made to feel welcome the moment we walked in the door. It was overwhelming, the extent of options and knowledge available.

Going to the implant center for the first time was scary and exciting. Hearing the details of the surgery is unnerving, but knowing that your child will hear is a miracle.

We had met the director of the [implant] center previously, so our first visit to the center was not strange, uncomfortable, or anxiety-provoking. In fact, we felt we were taking a very positive step with the support of wonderful, caring professionals.

We were nervous and very excited. We hoped that Grace would be a candidate. The entire experience was very informative and reassuring. The staff ... was wonderful.

First time I went, I met a ten-year-old girl with an implant. The mother spoke to the girl with her back turned and the girl understood her. I was very impressed.

Before our son's first implant, we visited three implant centers. The first one ... was too far from our home to consider using for the actual implant, but we just wanted to discuss implants in general with the CI surgeon there, and he was very helpful. At the second implant center ... we visited extensively with the audiologist ... and the CI surgeon. Both were very patient and helpful and took considerable time answering the numerous questions we had. ...We were also pleased that the audiologist provided us with a list of around thirty families of children who had been implanted there, and we called up many of these families to learn of their experiences with this center.... At the third center, the CI surgeon gave us a quick five-minute talk about cochlear implants ... and seemed quite startled when we asked him if he'd mind answering a few questions....When it came time to get the reimplant, we looked for an implant center that had considerable experience with reimplanting.

Which Device Should We Choose?

When our daughter received her implant, there were only two manufacturers to choose from. The first thing we did was compare current technology. Our next ... concern was service. We had so many equipment problems with hearing aids and FMs, so service was a big deciding factor. We called and e-mailed both companies with questions at various times and noted the response rate as well as the concern/effort that was taken with each request. Finally, we spoke with parents whose children were implanted with either manufacturer's device and asked similar questions so that we could weigh which company would best suit our needs.

[The device you choose] depends on the audiologist, therapist, and implant center you will be using. Ongoing support is key. The implant is the start of the process.

We had no choice for the first one. But when Louie was sixteen years old, he was reimplanted. Again, we had no choice because the Clarion was not available yet, so we accepted the Nucleus 22. I had heard and read good things about the Clarion, but I guess we will never really know which would have been better.

At the time, only the Nucleus 22 had been FDA-approved. There was not any question when deciding which one to get.

The Clarion was made of porcelain and seemed to be easily damaged if my son was accidentally hit in that area. Therefore, I chose the Nucleus 24.

At the time, the Nucleus 22 was available to children [and was] recommended by professionals. It was May, 1993 at Matt's time of implantation.

The choice was easy since our doctor only implanted the Nucleus 24.

The Nucleus 24 was the most advanced, with twenty-four available channels as opposed to twenty-two. Also, the Nucleus 24 has more options than the Clarion from our perspective.

This was a very difficult decision. At the time Jeremy was to be implanted, everyone had a Nucleus. We were being pushed by other parents to follow along. Clarion had just come out. Their results were amazing.

There was no alternative to the Nucleus 22 for a child at the time our son was implanted.

When I saw both the Nucleus 22 and Clarion, I found out that the Nucleus was planning on an ear-level processor eventually, so I decided on the Nucleus.

For our son's implant, we looked at all the pros and cons of the Clarion and the Nucleus 24, visited three different implant centers, and asked a great number of questions to each surgeon and audiologist.

What Did Family and Friends Say about the Implant?

Unless you are directly involved with raising a deaf child, for the most part, most people (yes, even family) don't understand. Everyone was very concerned we were looking for a miracle. Our family was concerned we were going to be in for another letdown. In our case, friends were more supportive than family. Even many of the local professionals raised their eyebrows at our decision.

It was our decision and no one else's. We are going to raise our son—not them. Since it was decided, then it's been a process of education, education, education and results, results, results!

This has proved to be one of the most difficult parts of our experience. People who don't know about CIs seem to have one of two different responses: Either they are skeptical about the implant, or they wonder if your child can really hear at all. Part of your role as a parent now involves educating others (i.e., my child is still hearing-impaired, he's still learning to use this device, the cochlear implant is a tool not a cure, etc.), and it's essential to educate those who are important in your child's life. But sometimes the best policy is just to ignore stupid comments—there are always going to be some people who just don't get it.

I didn't have any problems with this. We had read everything we could get our hands on about the device and what to expect—both times. We did not try to build anyone's hopes up for either device, but I must admit that I thought the second device would be much more effective than I think it has been.

All our families are from Brazil. Although my sister-in-law is deaf, she only became deaf at age four. From the beginning when Cristina was diagnosed, there was a lot to explain about the avenues we were taking on educating her . . . Cristina's use of sign language was never well understood by our family. It also had isolated them from communicating with her. Only the few more outgoing relatives tried to engage in a longer conversation with her during the times we came for vacation. We could sense that the cochlear implant would be very welcome by all our family. Our friends here were divided between those who thought Cristina should have the opportunity to learn how to listen and to communicate independently and those who felt that we were robbing her from her right to be deaf and to live among the deaf without a sense of having a disability.

I didn't tell relatives and friends until after my decision was made. I felt it was a decision I had to make for my child without influence.

We wanted our son to have the best opportunities he could have in life. The cochlear implant gave him what so far technology can give. Our families were open and knew they too were now part of a new world.

We were very excited, although most people didn't understand what we were talking about.

They supported us in our decision.

When we discussed this with our parents, they were supportive of the plans to receive an implant for our son. They wanted the chance to be able to communicate with their grandson desperately.

Everyone had a different reaction. Some said, "Go for it." Some said, "Are you sure?" There were a lot of questions, and we didn't have all the answers.

I spoke with my sister in Italy. She told me she also saw the implant on Italian TV and she felt it was a good decision.

What Were the Expectations
for the Initial Switch-On?

Since our child was implanted at a later age (almost five), my expectations were low. I wasn't sure how she would respond to sounds or voices. Our center told us each child responds differently. Our daughter had minimal reactions (no crying, no smiles, no wide eyes), until we got outside the hospital and heard the wonderful environmental sounds of New York City.

These expectations were clearly and realistically spelled out by the people at the implant center. . . . I also read a couple of books by people who had received implants and spoke to a couple of parents. But the experience was extremely emotional for us and our son. It's like giving birth: You can read about it, listen to stories told by other women, but nothing matches the actual experience.

We only expected safety sounds with the first device; so in three months, when Louie started using his voice and trying to talk, we were really delighted and surprised. We had been using Cued Speech with him as a communication mode, and he cued and mouthed back to us all the time. His receptive language was right on target for a hearing child, but we had some difficulties understanding him because his expressive [language] was too advanced for our Cued Speech reading abilities. This caused him frustration because his parents were too slow at understanding him. When sounds started to emerge with his cues and mouth movements, the field opened up very quickly and we were up and running.

Well ... looking back at that day, I find it really funny. I expected that once stimulated, Cristina would like what she was getting and become an enthusiastic participant in learning more about it like she had been when learning new signs or learning to read. Another parent that happened to be at the cochlear implant center that day told me how happy her daughter was when she was first fit with the speech processor. So, I was ready with a camera waiting for the grand moment.

I expected him to pick up where he left off. But it's been one-and-a-half years, and he is just picking up on the single words. I think I was expecting a miracle.

We were thoroughly briefed about what to expect, but we have it all on videotape.

We were well prepared and we actually didn't expect much. Our daughter did not react well and we were prepared. We had realistic expectations.

We thought Spencer would be very quiet and inquisitive and maybe an element of surprise.

We didn't know what to expect. We were praying for a miracle. We were looking forward to seeing a look of surprise on his face.

We don't remember our initial expectations. There was a fear that he might not respond to familiar words, such as his name.

We hoped for some response. We got a look of surprise and a little cry, then mommy cried!

I expected Giova to cry and say she heard me!

Since we had read of the varied responses a child has at the initial fitting, we had no preconceptions about how he would react.

What Was the Reaction to the Actual Switch-On?

I will never forget the first night we went home (Grandma's house). [M]y mother-in-law rang a bell and our daughter's eyes became wide. At that point, she clasped the bell, went into a corner (away from the noise) and rang the bell over and over again with a beautiful smile to show her sense of accomplishment! There were tears in all of our eyes. We knew our journey into sound was just beginning. It took about three to four weeks before she began to recognize her name and names of family members.

Our son looked surprised, puzzled, scared, and cried himself to sleep. There wasn't a dry eye in the house, which included extended family members and nannies. I felt happy and scared at the same time. I kept thinking, "I hope we did the right thing!"

We could see Alex went through different emotions in very quick succession: mild curiosity, confusion, and fear followed by five minutes of crying. Then, just as quickly, he was over it and was running around as if nothing had happened. He's now mapped at a volume level much higher than the one that made him cry just two weeks ago. He's adjusted very quickly.

I have it on grainy videotape, and when I come across the tape during clean-up around the house and slip it into the machine for a look back, I can remember it as if it was ten minutes ago (not nineteen years ago). He was so cute at three years old, and he was playing with blocks, and all of a sudden, he grabbed his ear and looked at me. I cued to him that he had just heard a sound. I cued the sounds of speech he was hearing. He was interested but continued to play. I, on the other hand, could not shut up.

Silvia, Cristina's older sister, was there too, participating in the game of dropping blocks in a bucket when she heard a sound. Well, I was ready, but Cristina had no facial reaction to sound at all. She was not excited, scared, or anything! Nothing! Well, I was hoping for something a lot more emotional in nature. Later, Cristina explained to me that she was "paying a lot of attention" to what she was getting.

He didn't appear to respond at all.

Our son sat on his daddy's lap. And when he first *felt* the sound, he hid his face in his daddy's chest. We, of course, were moved to tears.

Matt was overwhelmed at lunch immediately following the tune-up, and I remember [he] was frightened by the sound of traffic outside of the hospital. We felt thrilled he could hear, even if he was afraid.

Our daughter climbed into our laps and cried. We were, of course, disappointed but not daunted.

Spencer cried and cried and cried. He cried so loud; and the more he cried, the more he was afraid. We all remained quiet and spoke in whispers. We held Spencer tightly and gave him our physical reassurances.

Jeremy was very surprised. He cried at first. I think he was overwhelmed. They asked us to call his name. He turned around. Someone asked him if he wanted "one more," and he said, "One more." We cried tears of joy.

When the audiologist covered her mouth and said, "Matthew," he responded by saying, "Magew," which was how he pronounced his name at the time (age two). I was relieved and thrilled that he recognized his name.

She looked up, looked at us, and started to cry. We knew she heard something.

She got pale and didn't say anything. I felt I couldn't talk. I was so excited and scared.

At the initial tune-up, he cried some. At the initial tune-up after reimplantation, he didn't cry; instead he seemed startled at the new sounds he was hearing and appeared so affected by this that, during the tune-up, his voicing went silent. We knew the initial tune-up was just the first step in the process, so we didn't have all our hopes tied up in how he reacted then.

How Does the Implant Affect Communication within the Family?

During the first year, we saw so many changes. We had used Cued Speech since our daughter was two and continued to use it to feed her as much language as possible. What a joy when I called her from the other room and asked her what she wanted for lunch, and she responded appropriately! I am so thankful every time we carry on a conversation in the car. Some of our son's friends were seeing her become more vocal and actually understood her! Both friends and family were more at ease about communication with her.

One year later, our family communicates drastically differently. We are stricter with our son and the rest of the family about taking turns, listening, communicating constantly, relying less on television and more on reading . . . storytelling . . . roleplaying. It has forced us to all participate and communicate more, and we are all gaining from the experience!

Because of the combination of Cued Speech and the implant, Louie did not have any specific language delay. He enjoyed four years of Spanish and two years of French. He is taking Thai now in college.

When we found out that Cristina was profoundly deaf, we not only changed the language used at home, but we also added another "foreign" language: sign language.

All of us went to classes, including Silvia, our older daughter. Among other feelings, we were overwhelmed by this enterprise and its urgency. Communication was not concentrated in its contents, but we all had to put a lot of effort in its format. It had always been very important that Cristina also become aware of her environment, so I was always "directing" her attention to this and that around her. After she started to become a more comfortable user of the implant, we also noticed that we relied on Cristina to be responsible for her safety in busy areas, as well as become a greater participant in family conversations. My husband uses very little sign language with Cristina now. Her sister uses sign language when she has privacy in mind. I do the same. When visiting a place when the speaker is addressing a large group, I become Cristina's interpreter.

The cochlear implant allows us the choice of communicating through sign or verbal language.

We treat our son like a normal hearing child. We communicate "our" family way. He is responding beautifully. The implant allows our family to speak, listen, and react.

We communicate so much as a hearing family with the implant that we forget that Matt would not hear us enter the room without it.

Our daughter has always been in an Auditory-Verbal program, so our day-to-day therapy and involvement has not changed. However, the ease of our conversation is off the charts. There is no comparison to the hearing aids!

It has enhanced his relationships with grandparents and aunts and uncles. Spencer does not feel "left out" during conversations with family. He can also tell them what's on his mind.

A lot of times, it's easy to forget Jeremy is deaf. If we're downstairs and he's upstairs, we can call him and he answers. We can ask him questions from different rooms and he answers. We're amazed.

Immeasurably. Prior to the implant, there was a great deal of frustration and mind reading. As the years have unfolded, we are able to communicate fairly normally in the oral mode.

The implant affected family communication 100 percent. Grace's receptive and expressive language grow daily.

It changed our family a lot. She used a lot of sign language before. Now, little by little, she doesn't point anymore. We also spoke only in Italian before, but now we speak more English.

Did the Implant Change the Communication Methodology in Use Before Surgery?

In order to maximize the potential of the implant, we have tried to provide our daughter with as much auditory stimuli as possible. We have also tried to place her in environments where she will gain access to language, but not be too overwhelmed with noise. We only use Cued Speech in noisy environments to explain new concepts or in situations where she is not wearing the external processor, such as pool time.

We are committed to the oral/spoken method and whatever it takes to be successful. We implement therapy in a playful manner most of the time. We are strict about using the implant from the moment he wakes up to the moment he goes to bed. All members of the family and our nanny try to be in sync with what is being implemented at therapy. We try to achieve a good balance between letting our son be a child and the constant learning process.

I can't imagine not going for some concept of sound if it is available. I know that some proponents hang on to the belief that a deaf child has the right to stay deaf, and I can only tell them that, at least with the implant, the deaf child has the choice. Without it, the child has no choice.

Cristina is now sixteen years old. Initially, I made the decision as to how strict I was going to be to have her switch from using a visual language to using voice and listening. For her to have the opportunity to learn to listen, I had the family engage in using techniques based on the Auditory-Verbal approach. We covered our mouths when speaking and reduced the background noise to allow her to learn how to process language auditorily. As she became a more comfortable listener and speaker, she also got older and had her own ideas as to how she wanted things to be for her. She enjoys being with other people her age and being able to freely communicate with them using voice. In the classroom, she likes to use the sign language interpreter. At home, after a busy day at school, she may take a break from the implant. She uses voice to communicate, and I may sign for accuracy since lighting does affect how well she can lipread.

With the implant, I thought he would not need sign, but he uses both.

We are aware of the implant and inform others so JQ can get the maximum communication from others. Others are very respectful and are always impressed to see how well JQ is doing.

I am a true supporter of the oral approach to deafness and a realist that it is a hearing world. I believe the implant is a tool, such as eyeglasses.

AV Therapy meant we haven't changed much.

Communication on any level promotes and can sustain relationships. Barriers to communication make us uncomfortable and without friendships. The cochlear implants give people communication tools to build relationships with.

We're strong believers in the oral approach. The implant has given Jeremy the ability to develop age-appropriate speech and language. He is happy to be able to communicate with his friends, sing, etc.

We have always felt strongly that we wanted our son to communicate orally. The implant has enabled him to do so quite effectively.

Grace wears her implant from the time she gets up in the morning until bedtime. We try to treat her like a normal hearing child.

When she was one-and-a-half years old, we placed her in a school where she learned sign language. She couldn't communicate verbally very well. When she turned nine years old and got the implant, many things changed. We went to a different school and stopped sign language.

With an implant that works, communication via spoken English is very achievable—given adequate follow-up.

What Kind of Educational Services
Does a Child with an Implant Typically Receive?

The first year and a half of her implant use was wonderful. We were fortunate to have a speech-language pathologist who aggressively investigated and learned the various ways to maximize the implant's use. The cochlear implant is a fairly new concept in our community. Many professionals do not understand its potential and the need for continued auditory work and language development. Although it has been a struggle, our daughter has still made considerable progress. Most parents' vision and expectations are higher than what school districts can and will provide for rehabilitation of the cochlear implant.

I hold to the belief that there are parents who research and think and work to bring sensible smart language opportunities to their child and that there are parents that do not have a clue how language is developed and expect the schools and the device to perform some kind of magic. That day may be coming, but we did not have that luxury. We moved to get what we thought was the best education for our son. I am not lamenting because I'm proud of Louie's progress. I have seen others go farther and I've seen others do less.

Although we do not live in a small town, there is certainly a predominant way to approach the education of the profoundly deaf students here. From the beginning, we have found that services could be easily found if we agreed with the philosophy of Simultaneous Communication. Although we ended up signing with Cristina, we could not have found services if we did not agree with embracing this approach. Later, after the implant, we have struggled to have what we called appropriate services delivered in school. Unfortunately, we were more in the position of "groundbreakers" [rather] than that of [parents] receiving support for what we believed Cristina needed. Taking into consideration that she has Usher's Syndrome, we continue to experience resistance in providing certain types of services for her. As we envision Cristina going to college in two years, we have already started to look at how well different institutions are able to provide a variety of services to their students with hearing impairments and combined disabilities. Cristina has always been an honor student and, although this fact opened a lot of opportunities for her, the success of her programming has oftentimes been evaluated by her grades and not by her needs.

We are in the process of mainstreaming our three-year-old. I'll have to let you know about this later.

Services were obtained through our local school intermediate unit but were not sufficient to provide all educational objectives. Therefore, Matt had many additional hours of tutoring on a parent-provided basis.

The implant center . . . has been Spencer's greatest educational asset. Along with that foundation, the team at the local school has been more than accommodating, forming an alliance with the implant specialists.

Getting services requires *a lot* of patience and persistence. Our district is now setting up a special division for children with implants so they can get therapists trained in this field.

Our son has always been mainstreamed, and we have enjoyed a good working relationship with our district. For the most part, we have been able to secure the services we felt he needed.

We now have her mainstreamed in a resource room. She receives speech therapy and is seen by a teacher of the deaf.

How Does a Child with an Implant Relate to Other Deaf Children?

Our daughter plays with another girl who is deaf, but she is being raised orally. So they both communicate orally. Although she has been around deaf children who use Cued Speech expressively, she does not use Cued Speech to communicate. Our daughter also has a hearing friend whose parents are deaf, and when they are together, they choose to communicate by signing. With signing deaf peers, she tries very hard to read the deaf child's lips and understand the signs being used. It is our intention to have our daughter take an ASL class when she is older to help her better communicate with other deaf peers.

Our son is still too young (three years old) to even have relationships. But we do plan to have him try to develop relationships with kids who are deaf (especially those with implants), so that he has the support of friends who share common experiences.

Louie had buddies in the Cued Speech division of auditory services during grade school. He has been fully mainstreamed since kindergarten with a Cued Speech transliterator for all his classes. But when he reached junior high, the three divisions of the school program were lumped together in the same school, and that's when he developed some unhappy memories. The signing kids made fun of him and the signing staff were overtly rude about Cued Speech and the implant. During his second year of senior high, Louie decided he wanted to be in his home school, where he would be the only deaf person. He felt that the deaf were clumped together as a group by the hearing kids in the school he was attending. He transferred out and seemed to be much happier. He was reimplanted the beginning of his senior year. He chose ASI in Phoenix for his university and is heavily into airway science and airport management. He has made no deaf friends since the time of junior high and only retained a few from then.

[In the child's own words] Well, I have to tell truthfully, unlike some other children with cochlear implants, I grew up submerged in the Deaf culture. I was educated . . . by sign language up to age eight, two years after I received my cochlear implant. I had a very close relationship with a circle of deaf friends when I was little, and I continue to keep in touch with them to this date. I have a unique friendship with them and I continue to cherish them.

From the time Cristina was very little, she liked to play with hearing children. One deaf boy has been her friend since they were one-and-a-half years old. She has also developed a strong friendship with another oral deaf girl. But mostly, her strongest friendships have been with students from gifted programs that she has been involved with along the years, and none of them is deaf.

Plays well. Limited communication.

He has five children he has been friends with since he was first identified. I don't think JQ really knows he can't hear.

He does not know any deaf children.

She is and has always been mainstreamed. We try to get her play dates with other deaf children because she knows she is different from her hearing peers. She wants to hear like her friends. We feel it's important for her to have children with implants as role models.

Spencer only knows one other deaf person, and that person is very inquisitive about Spencer's device.

Spencer continues to use Simultaneous Communication no matter who he is with.

Jeremy treats everyone the same. We never labeled him or his friends, so he doesn't see any difference.

He enjoyed meeting other children with the implant last year [summer of 1999] when he participated in a research study at CID. He knows several deaf children from going to the League for the Hard of Hearing but rarely sees them anymore.

Grace acts like a normal hearing child and treats all children the same.

Now she doesn't know any other deaf children.

Our son is very outgoing around other children, whether deaf or hearing, and gets along well with them.

How Does a Child with an Implant Relate to Hearing Children?

Our daughter has been mainstreamed for two years and most of her friends are hearing. Early on, I had to be part of the playgroup to make sure she understood the conversation. Now, the girls go off and play without me having to be present all the time. With her close friends, if she doesn't understand what they say initially, she asks them to repeat themselves. Also, in many cases, the hearing playmate realizes she missed something, so they rephrase it for her. These are some wonderful skills both children are learning on their own!

Right now, most of our son's playmates are hearing children because of proximity, distance, and age. Also, his older sister is his best friend, and he goes to a mainstream preschool. Whether it is a coincidence or not, his social skills and interaction with others have flourished since he got his implant.

Louie found that he could make friends on the Internet with people who didn't know he was hearing-impaired. He found that the foreign children in high school and college are far more patient and friendly to a person like him that is considered hard of hearing (because of the implant). They speak more slowly . . . simply because English is not their first language. Louis does not avoid communication with anyone that is placed in his environment. He especially enjoys the people he works with at his summer and holiday break job at Dulles Airport in Virginia. He is a ramp agent and works on several of the international flights.

[In the child's own words] Even before my implant was installed, I had good relationships with hearing children. I've always found it comfortable communicating with them and haven't encountered many problems in my fifteen years. I've always been able to develop rapport with hearing children with ease, but, of course, there have been hearing children who have been resistant about my deafness, but these are comparatively rare.

Plays well but very limited communication.

He has several friends outside of his therapy group that he interacts with. He learns a lot from his eight-year-old sister.

He has been extremely social and out-going and has been fortunate to have been with several friends since kindergarten in their social group. Now he is a high school senior. He is branching out at basketball camps with others and through community service work. He seems to make friends easily with hearing peers.

All her friends are hearing children. Initially, her hearing loss was an issue because her speech was unclear. Now that's becoming less of an issue.

Spencer continues to use Simultaneous Communication no matter who he is with, although he tends to use very little sign when with his schoolmates and friends. They can understand Spencer more each day. Spencer's friends have never singled him out or made issue with his implant. If anything, they are protective of him.

He has always been fully mainstreamed, and his best friends have normal hearing. He rather enjoys his position of being special, of being the only one. However, from kindergarten until spring of second grade, he did not like being different or having a cochlear implant. After seeing Caitlin Parton on "60 Minutes," he did an about-face and proudly presented his implant to his second grade class. Since then, he has explained the device to this third grade class and subsequently to his bunkmates at camp. Recently, he very spontaneously kissed me on the cheek and said, "Thank you for getting me a cochlear implant." During this time period, he has also expanded his friendships and has really blossomed socially. With his greater acceptance of his "difference," has come great self-assurance.

She talks on the phone and plays with only hearing children. In a special summer program this year, there were five children, and she became good friends with them in only twenty days! All hearing children.

What Is an Implanted Child's Perception of His or Her Own Deafness?

Our daughter considered herself deaf before the implant. Today, she asks me not to yell at her because she's not deaf!

Our son is too young still. He doesn't seem to notice a difference between him and others.

Louie seems to be of the attitude that his deafness is an inconvenience, not a culture or lifestyle. We, as his parents, never felt sorry for him or let him feel sorry for himself. He has a dynamite sense of humor and is one of the most talkative and gregarious persons in or out of our family. He is far more adventurous than we would like him to be. He has traveled many times to Japan, France, and Thailand on his own, starting at the age of sixteen, for months at a time.

Cristina herself had questions about the outcome of the surgery. She was six years old at the time. . . . She asked me, "Mom, after the implant, will I be hearing or deaf?" I told her, "You will be both! Hearing when you have your implant on, and deaf when you have your implant off." We talked for a long time that night about what it meant to hear, and what her silence meant to her so far. We talked about being able to expect things to show up in front of you because you "heard it coming." We continued having these conversations for all these years since she has had her implant. About eight years after she had had the implant, I was amazed that Cristina did not know that not everybody heard everything all the time. She thought that if you had hearing, you heard everything, and that distance, accent, [and] background noise only affected people with a hearing loss! Why did it take us so long to talk about that?

I don't know.

I'm not sure if he knows he can't hear. He knows the device allows him to hear. He wants it on.

Matthew feels hard of hearing, not deaf. I think he feels he is part of the hearing world and can do whatever hearing people do, with greater effort and hard work.

She realizes that she hears differently from her friends, and she is beginning to express feelings of wanting to hear like her friends.

Spencer's current perception at seven years of age is "I can't hear that. I need my implant on." He does not see himself as different. He is just Spencer.

Jeremy is very accepting of his deafness. We never told him he was deaf. We explained the problem with his ears, the surgery, other people's handicap, etc. We did have one rough time when he started crying about not wanting to wear his implant, but we explained that he's lucky there was something that could be done about it and that the technology is always changing. He likes to hear about the latest changes and is looking forward to his BTE. It is heartbreaking to discuss, but we're glad he has such a positive attitude.

He likes being special.

She does not think she is different at all. She is very outgoing.

She feels that she isn't deaf anymore. Now she is hearing. Before she couldn't hear people call her or talk on the phone. Now she can. She also says she used to not have any "ideas;" now she has ideas for what's happening around her.

He loves to show his headpiece and speech processor to everyone he meets. He recognizes his own situation when we read cochlear implant storybooks to him.

What Were Some Unanticipated Benefits from the Implant?

The implant has superseded my original expectations. At first, I just wanted her to be able to hear environmental sounds that could pose danger to her. Secretly, I yearned for her to someday say, "Mom, I love you." She has accomplished all this and more and continues to greatly benefit from the implant and the new programming software as it is introduced.

We did not expect how the whole family would gain from his experience with the implant: the celebrations of every word he utters, the pride felt for his accomplishments, and the unity it has brought our family.

The fact that our son started to speak after remaining silent from the day he lost his hearing at eleven months of age until he was implanted at the age of three-and-a-half years of age will always remain the most pleasant surprise of my life.

When we first thought about a cochlear implant for Cristina, we were struggling to have her become aware of her own voice and to be able to anticipate dangerous situations when by herself in the streets and in parking lots. Of course, as that happened naturally in the first few months after implantation, our expectations were that she developed enough listening skills so we could call her at a short distance instead of having to tap her to call her attention. Then, we thought she could understand what we wanted to tell her. Then, she could talk to us using simple words. Then, we wanted her to become a listener and speaker of her own. Then, she went to Miami, Aruba, and Brazil on her own, and we wanted her to be able to communicate in Spanish and Portuguese (which she did!). She does remind us that it all takes effort, and she is not always able to be putting 100 percent of effort into this. Her daily life has to require a "reasonable" amount of energy from her. Listening and speaking is how she gets to the things she really wants (like relationships and academics), but we should not lose sight that this is the *how*, and the really important things [are] the *what* she has determined to get. In other words, if listening takes up all she has to give, the goal in itself may never be achieved since she would have exhausted her resources just to get there.

Each day JQ learns a little bit more, and he expresses himself a little bit more. It brings great joy to his daddy and me.

At the time of implantation, we were hoping for any degree of help from the device. Unanticipated benefits were the degree [to which] Matt could understand open-set speech.

While not exactly unanticipated, it should be noted that the implant has completely transformed our daughter from a behavior and social standpoint. Many of her improper, antisocial behaviors are disappearing.

Spencer can hear birds and aircraft. He *still*, after three years, says, "What's that?" He enjoys TV more and is beginning to like music. He can keep a beat!

We never thought we'd be able to call Jeremy from a different floor and get a response. He's talking on the phone. He knows all the Pokemon characters. He's just like everybody else.

The whole experience has been a joy. We never expected it to be this great. Grace communicates very well. She is a happy well-adjusted child.

She can hear me from another room and comprehend what I've said and answers me. She feels so comfortable now. She looks much more relaxed. She says she isn't embarrassed or nervous anymore.

The implant allows us to give [our son] more freedom of movement [so] he doesn't have to be right next to us to hear what we say or to warn him of dangers.

What Do You Wish You Knew Then That You Know Now?

The technology is moving so fast. There are things you learn on a daily basis. There are always things we feel we wish we had known, but we are glad we proceeded with the information available at the time and look forward to the future with great anticipation.

I wish I had become a member of CICircle and turned to a "support group" earlier on, because you keep going and forget about the importance of emotional support from others ... who are going through (or have gone through) what you are going through. Also, the lessons learned by others are so crucial to taking shortcuts.

To prepare for the surgery, buy some shirts or pajamas that button down the front so you don't have to worry about pulling clothes over a bandaged head. Call the children's ward at the hospital ahead of time and ask if they have a TV and VCR on wheels available, which you can park next to the bed. If so, take all your child's favorite videos. Take some extra pillows and blankets (for you and for the child), and don't forget to take extra clothes for yourself because you don't know what may happen to the clothes you are wearing. Most of all, this can be a very stressful time so be good to yourself.

I wish I had known that some places are better than others at getting the mapping more accurate. I feel for the first two years or so with the new implant that Louie did not fully understand that he had to work more with it and push its capacity to get more and better sounds. He was satisfied with so little because he was so used to the single-channel device.

When Cristina first got her implant, my main questions were in relation of what to expect of her. I wanted to know what would the "natural" sequence of skills that she should be acquiring be, and how to evaluate her performance when helping her. I wanted to know more about her limitations. Now, I can tell when the listening situation is too difficult for her; but in the beginning, I did not know that since she never showed signs of detecting any sounds before the implant.

I was very informed by everyone from the very beginning.

I wish I knew then that Matt would be entering his senior year of high school as an honor student, on the telephone more and more, and enjoying outdoor summer concerts.

It just may take six months of therapy and repeated word usage before your son or daughter begins using prepositions. But then, one night, she'll say, "Mommy, I want to sleep next to you."...and you'll let her!

I would have implanted her at a much younger age, as soon as possible. I never would have put her in a school for the deaf. I would have mainstreamed her when she was in kindergarten.

We are profoundly sorry that our son was not diagnosed from birth. What a tragic waste of years. We would have contacted the implant center immediately had we been given that chance.

I wish I knew how normal life would be. I wish I knew life was going to get easier, happier....When you first hear the news, it's devastating. I think people should set very high expectations for their children. Getting Jeremy to where he is now has been the hardest thing we have ever done. He has *really* worked hard....A lot of time, blood, sweat, and tears must be put into making it work but it's worth it.

I wish I knew how wonderful it would turn out. It would have really helped on the day of the surgery.

In the final analysis, parenting a child with a cochlear implant requires certain adaptations to generally accepted parenting skills. It may be easy to lose sight of the larger parenting issues in light of the specific needs of a child with a hearing loss *and* a cochlear implant. In order to encourage parents to consider the "big picture," we close with the following thoughts on parenting.

The Millennial Parent

What is the best way to parent? How do we become good parents? The answers to these questions are the subject of talk shows, books, magazine articles, interviews, websites, and weekly support groups. One would think that with all of that attention, we, as a society, would have definitive answers by now. If the truth be known, there are as many answers to these questions as there are parents and children. The present generation of parents barely resembles the generation that preceded them. In all probability, the previous generation felt the same way about their parents. What hasn't really changed, however, is the fact that parents want what is best for their children. What actually *is* best and *how* it is obtained, is what creates the differences in parenting styles and ultimately in child achievement.

Parents today, as in the past, come in all sizes, shapes, and colors. Families, however, have evolved from the traditional, married, nuclear unit with a working father, stay-at-home mother, and children to many different configurations. Now, more children than ever before are raised by dual working parents, single parents, joint custody parents, alternative lifestyle partners, or even grandparents. This diversity brings new and exciting changes to society but also creates challenges that need to be overcome in order to fulfill the goals of good parenting. Instead of the home becoming the center of family activity, it is more often a pit stop in the frenetic race towards the next appointment. Family members carry beepers, cell phones, and electronic organizers in order to keep themselves on track and to communicate with one another. Traditionalists look at this behavior and shrug disapprovingly, yet many parents consider technology a blessing. Regardless of one's perspective on this techno-craze, there is no going back. Some parents may stand firm in their fight for a simpler, easier family life, but, in all likelihood, children will discover and embrace technology on their own.

Dealing with the technology of the age certainly presents its trials and tribulations for those parenting in the twenty-first century. Whether for entertainment or education, children can now converse with other children halfway around the globe through e-mail, and they can access information through the Internet. Exposure to other cultures and societies can have a profound effect on the way children think. However, just as parents of the early twentieth century sat in the park to watch their children, ensuring that no harm would come to them, parents in today's era must also oversee their children's new technological activities to ensure their safety as well. This becomes difficult as "latchkey" children spend more time without supervision. But, parents who want the best for their children will learn what they must about technology and supervise its use to ensure their children's well-being.

In addition to coping with technology, however, parents must manage the ever-changing structure of the family. Extended families have become so over-extended that some children may have more than one set of "parents" to whom they report. Full-time caregivers may spend more time with children than working parents. Also, in some households, it is not unusual for the new "sandwich" generation to be caring for young children and elderly parents all under the same roof. Supervision of children therefore may be the responsibility of several individuals instead of the traditional two parents. When competing child-rearing philosophies collide, children receive mixed signals and become confused and disillusioned.

Societal pressures have created volcano-like situations that are awaiting eruption. With a mounting emphasis on education and a drive for money and stature, competition for children to achieve the best grades and get into the best schools has never been fiercer. The effort to improve and strengthen education is a respectable goal. The only question becomes how much this goal is achieved at the expense of the child's psyche. Preschools are adding computers to their classrooms so that their three-year-olds can get a head start on other children. More school systems are introducing world languages at the elementary level. Children in high school are enrolled in college-level courses. Many parents believe that these types of adaptations, which expand their children's knowledge base at earlier stages in their education, are in the best interests of their children. In some circumstances, they may be correct. In some cases, they are not; however, parents are much more vocal now than at any time in the past about their views on education and their children's needs. They have learned to be advocates for their children, and they work to create the best educational environment.

Schools are beginning to feel the pressure as well. Parents are more vocal with their views on education and their children's needs. They have learned to be advocates for their children to ensure that the best educational environment is created. Education is perceived as a prized commodity by most families. The value placed on education has grown logarithmically through the years as more parents have achieved higher educational levels. Parents with knowledge yield the power to implement change when systems fail. Parents who are passive find a system that easily conforms to their idleness.

The final mission of parenting involves letting go. Parents who have pushed, prodded, worried, and fretted about the success of their children will find that there comes a time when they must accept their children for who they are (or who they are not) and release them to the world. A parent's success in this endeavor may be linked to the degree of independence afforded the child during his or her development. Fostering independence, however, should never be mistaken with leaving a child unsupervised. Children who become independent thinkers are provided with the right amount of nurturing, goal setting, limit setting, and support. Calculating exactly those amounts is the reason for the talk shows, books, magazine articles, interviews, websites, and weekly support groups on parenting.

Final Thoughts

Like all decisions made for children when they are young, only the passage of time can validate the parents' choice to implant their child. Regardless of the ultimate benefit obtained for any given child with an implant, parents who make an informed decision can take comfort in the fact that they approached implantation with as much information as possible. It is our hope that this book will become one of the many resources available to parents to guide them as they consider the appropriateness of implant technology for their child with hearing loss.

Appendix A

NAD Position Statement on Cochlear Implants

The National Association of the Deaf (NAD) is an education and advocacy organization committed to promotion, protection, and preservation of the rights and quality of life of deaf and hard of hearing individuals in the United States of America. The targeted audience for this paper includes parents of deaf children, deaf individuals, medical professionals, and the media.

The NAD recognizes that diversity within the deaf community itself, and within the deaf experience, has not been acknowledged or explained very clearly in the public forum. Deafness is diverse in its origin and history, in the adaptive responses made to it, and in the choices that deaf adults and parents of deaf children continue to make about the ever-increasing range of communication and assistive technology options. Diversity requires mutual respect for individual and/or group differences and choices.

The NAD welcomes all individuals regardless of race, religion, ethnic background, socioeconomic status, cultural orientation, mode of communication, preferred language use, hearing status, educational background, and use of technologies. The NAD also welcomes deaf, hard of hearing and hearing family members, educators, and other professionals serving deaf and hard of hearing children and adults.

The NAD subscribes to the wellness model upon which the physical and psychosocial integrity of deaf children and adults is based. The general public needs information about the lives of the vast majority of deaf and hard of hearing individuals who have achieved optimal adjustments in all phases of life, have well-integrated and healthy personalities, and have attained self-actualizing levels of functioning, all with or without the benefits of hearing aids, cochlear implants, and other assistive devices.

The NAD recognizes all technological advancements with the potential to foster, enhance, and improve the quality of life of all deaf and hard of hearing persons. During the past three decades, technological developments such as closed captioning, e-mail and the Internet, two-way pagers, text telephones, telecommunications relay services, video interpreting services, visual alerting devices, vibro-tactile devices, hearing aids, amplification devices, audio loop and listening systems have had an important role in leveling the playing field. The role of the cochlear implant in this regard is evolving and will certainly change in the future. Cochlear implants are not appropriate for *all* deaf and hard of hearing children and adults. Cochlear implantation is a technology that represents a tool to be used in some forms of communication, and not a cure for deafness. Cochlear implants provide sensitive hearing, but do not, by themselves, impart the ability to understand spoken language through listening alone. In addition, they do not guarantee the development of cognition or reduce the benefit of emphasis on parallel visual language and literacy development.

The NAD recognizes the rights of parents to make informed choices for their deaf and hard of hearing children, respects their choice to use cochlear implants and all other assistive devices, and strongly supports the development of the whole child and of language and literacy. Parents have the right to know about and understand the various options available, including all factors that might impact development. While there are some successes with implants, success stories should not be over-generalized to every individual.

Rationale: The focus of the 2000 NAD position statement on cochlear implants is on preserving and promoting the psychosocial integrity of deaf and hard of hearing children and adults. The adverse effects of inflammatory statements about the deaf population of this country must be addressed. Many within the medical profession continue to view deafness essentially as a disability and an abnormality and believe that deaf and hard of hearing individuals need to be "fixed" by cochlear implants. This pathological view must be challenged and corrected by greater exposure to and interaction with well-adjusted and successful deaf and hard of hearing individuals.

The media often describe deafness in a negative light, portraying deaf and hard of hearing children and adults as handicapped and second-class citizens in need of being "fixed" with cochlear implants. There is little or no portrayal of successful, well adjusted deaf and hard of hearing children and adults without implants. A major reason implantation and oral language training have been pursued so aggressively by the media, the medical profession, and parents is not simply because of the hoped-for benefits that come with being able to hear in a predominantly hearing society but more because of the perceived burdens associated with being deaf.

Because cochlear implant technology continues to evolve, to receive mainstream acceptance, and to be acknowledged as part of today's reality, it is urgent to be aware of and responsive to the historical treatment of deaf persons. This perspective makes it possible to provide more realistic guidelines for parents of deaf and hard of hearing children and for pre-lingually and post-lingually deafened adults.

Wellness Model: Many deaf and hard of hearing people straddle the "deaf and hearing worlds" and function successfully in both. There are many people with implants who use sign language and continue to be active members of the deaf community and who ascribe to deaf culture and heritage. There are many deaf and hard of hearing individuals, with and without implants, who are high-achieving professionals, talented in every imaginable career field. They, too, are successfully effective parents, raising well-adjusted deaf, hard of hearing and hearing children. As citizens, they continue to make contributions to improve the quality of life for society at large. Deaf and hard of hearing individuals throughout the ages have demonstrated psychological strength and social skills when surviving and overcoming society's misconceptions, prejudices, and discriminatory attitudes and behaviors, thus attesting to their resilience, intelligence, and integrity.

Given the general lack of awareness about the reality of the wellness model, the NAD strongly urges physicians, audiologists, and allied professionals to refer parents to qualified experts in deafness and to other appropriate resources so that parents can make fully informed decisions – that is, decisions that incorporate far more than just the medical-surgical. Such decisions involve language preferences and usage, educational placement and training opportunities, psychological and social development, and the use of technological devices and aids.

The Cochlear Implant: The most basic aspect of the cochlear implant is to help the user perceive sound, i.e., the sensation of sound that is transmitted past the damaged cochlea to the brain. In this strictly sensorineural manner, the implant works: the sensation of sound is delivered to the brain. The stated goal of the implant is for it to function as a tool to enable deaf children to develop language based on spoken communication.

Cochlear implants do not eliminate deafness. An implant is not a "cure" and an implanted individual is still deaf. Cochlear implants may destroy what remaining hearing an individual may have. Therefore, if the deaf or hard of hearing child or adult later prefers to use an external hearing aid, that choice may be removed.

Unlike post-lingually deafened children or adults who have had prior experience with sound comprehension, a pre-lingually deafened child or adult does not have the auditory foundation that makes learning a spoken language easy. The situation for those progressively deafened or suddenly deafened later in life is different. Although the implant's signals to the brain are less refined than those provided by an intact cochlea, an individual who is accustomed to receiving signals about sound can fill in certain gaps from memory. While the implant may work quite well for post-lingually deafened individuals, this result just cannot be generalized to pre-lingually deafened children for whom spoken language development is an arduous process, requiring long-term commitment by parents, educators, and support service providers, with no guarantee that the desired goal will be achieved.

Parents: Parents face challenges when their child is born deaf or becomes deaf. At least ninety percent of deaf and hard of hearing children are born to hearing parents who usually want their children to be like themselves, to understand sound, to use their voices and verbally express their thoughts through spoken language, and to hear the voices and spoken language of those around them.

However, language and communication are not the same as speech, nor should the ability to speak and/or hear be equated with intelligence, a sense of well-being and lifelong success. Communication and cognition are vital ingredients of *every* child's development, regardless of the mode in which it is expressed, i.e., visual or auditory.

Despite the pathological view of deafness held by many within the medical profession, parents would benefit by seeking out opportunities to meet and get to know successful deaf and hard of hearing children and adults who are fluent in sign language and English, both with and without implants. The NAD encourages parents and deaf adults to research other options besides implantation. If implantation is the option of choice, parents should obtain all information about the surgical procedure, surgical risks, post-surgical auditory and speech training requirements, and potential benefits and limitations so as to make informed decisions.

Cochlear implant surgery is a beginning, not an end. The surgery decision represents the beginning of a process that involves a long-term, and likely, life-long commitment to auditory training, rehabilitation, acquisition of spoken and visual language skills, follow-up, and possibly additional surgeries. Whatever choices parents make, the primary goal should be to focus on the "whole child" and early language development/literacy and cognitive development. The absence of visual language opportunities can result in developmental delays that can be extremely difficult to reverse. Since the first six years are critical for language acquisition and usage, concurrent acquisition of visual and written language skills should be stressed.

Further improvements to cochlear implant technology and greater experience with educating and supporting pre-lingually deafened children and adults may later result in better outcomes for both of these populations than are achieved at present. In the meantime, though, parents of deaf and hard of hearing children need to be aware that a decision to forego implantation for their children does not condemn their children to a world of meaningless silence. Regardless of whether or not a deaf or hard of hearing child receives an implant, the child will function within both the hearing and the deaf communities. For these reasons, parents of pre-lingually deaf children presently have a reasonable basis upon which to decline implantation for their child. Parents must feel comfortable with their decision, whether they choose implantation or not.

Once parents have arrived at a decision, they want their decision to be validated. They seek reassurances often solely from within the medical and professional hearing health care community. This is a serious and major concern to the NAD. By releasing this position statement, the NAD seeks to alert, educate, and inform parents about deafness and the deaf community.

Recommendations

The NAD hereby makes the following recommendations for action:

Professional Training: Medical professionals have historically been the first point of contact for parents of deaf children. Their expertise is valuable but is primarily limited only to their medical areas of expertise. They should *not* be viewed as, nor should they function as, experts with regard to larger issues such as the educational, psychological, social, and linguistic needs of the deaf child. Medical professionals may be experts regarding the mysteries of the inner ear, but they are *not* experts regarding the *inner* lives of deaf children and adults. Psychological, social, educational, cultural and communication aspects of deafness, including the wellness model, must be a significant part of every medical school curriculum, especially within the specialty of oto-laryngology. In-service training programs should be implemented for all interdisciplinary staff at cochlear implant centers that would include guidance and counseling methods with parents of deaf children and adults considering cochlear implants. These training programs should be con-ducted by professional counselors who are trained, qualified, and com-petent to work and communicate with deaf and hard of hearing children and adults and their families.

Early Assessment of Hearing Aid Benefit: It is widely under-stood and accepted that a trial period of hearing aid use is necessary prior to cochlear implantation. Advanced digital hearing aids should be explored. The NAD encourages that this effort be earnest and of appropriate duration for adequate assessment by objective testing and skilled observation of behaviors and communication skills. This assess-ment is complicated by the child's lack of prior auditory experience, and inability to communicate what s/he is hearing. The length of this trial period will vary with the individual. Further research by the medi-cal and educational communities regarding objective hearing assess-ment and hearing aid trials is strongly encouraged.

Cochlear Implant Team: Candidacy assessment and surgery must be performed in a medical setting that has a close working relationship with a team of professionals that will provide ongoing long-term support to implant recipients. To be a responsible implant center, caution must be taken when describing the potential benefits of implantation, includ-ing risks, limitations, and long-term implications. Parents of deaf chil-dren and adults must be assisted in developing realistic and appropriate expectations. Critical to both pediatric and adult cochlear implantation and the long-range medical, audiological, psychological, social, emotional, educational, and vocational adjustment is access to implant centers fully complemented by an interdisciplinary staff, including rehabilitation specialists, psychologists and counselors. Implant center personnel must also work with and involve deafness professionals in education and in the helping professions. It takes a coordinated team of specialists, parents, educators and counselors to raise an implanted child and to sup-port an implanted adult over an extended period of time. The implant team is also morally obligated to recognize when the implant experience has been unsuccessful and provide alternate strategies for language training.

Habilitation: An essential component of the cochlear implant process is habilitation. Parents and professionals must make a long-term commitment to integrating listening strategies throughout the child's day at home and at school. It is important to recognize that a newly implanted child is unable to understand spoken language through listening alone. Therefore parents and professionals should continue to use sign language to ensure age-appropriate psychological, social, cognitive, and language development.

Insurance Coverage: The NAD recommends that medical insurance carriers also provide fair and equitable coverage for hearing aid devices and associated support services.

Media: Reporters, journalists, anchors and directors of newspapers, television networks and film are encouraged to research and prepare their material more carefully and without bias. There is a serious need for a more balanced approach to fact-finding and reporting.

Research: Longitudinal research is critically needed, including a more thorough analysis of those for whom the implant is not working. Future research should involve highly controlled, manufacturer-independent and unbiased research on the long-term outcomes of childhood implants on auditory and communicative development, academic and intellectual development and achievement, psychological, social and emotional adjustment, and interpersonal relationship functioning. Comparative research on children without implants receiving parallel support services should also be conducted, especially those for whom sign language is the primary form of communication. Research findings relative to children with and without cochlear implants in educated lay terms must be made available and disseminated to deaf individuals, to parents of implanted children, to those in the helping professions, and to those contemplating implants.

Parents: The NAD knows that parents love and care deeply about their deaf children. Since the decision to perform implant surgery on the deaf child is made for the child, it is necessary for parents to become educated about cochlear implants – the potential benefits, the risks, and all the issues that they entail. During this critical education process, parents have both the need and the right to receive unbiased information about the pros and cons of cochlear implants and related matters. The NAD knows that parents want to make informed decisions. Parents also would benefit by opportunities to interact with successful deaf and hard of hearing adults, as well as with parents of deaf and hard of hearing children.

Deafness is irreversible. Even with the implant and increased sound perception, the child is still deaf. Cochlear implants are not a cure for deafness. The most serious parental responsibility from the very beginning is total commitment to, and involvement with, their child's overall development and well-being. Throughout the developmental years, the deaf child – implanted or not, mainstreamed or not – should receive education in deaf studies, including deaf heritage, history of deafness and deaf people, particularly stories and accounts of deaf people who have succeeded in many areas of life.

Support Services: Parents must understand that, after suitability testing and the decision-making process, the actual surgical procedure is just the beginning – a prelude to a lifetime proposition for the child and years of commitment by the parents. Implanted children are still deaf and will continue to require educational, psychological, audiological assessment, auditory and speech training, and language support services for a long period of time. Services for families and children should be provided in a manner that is consistent with standards set by the Individuals with Disabilities Education Act (IDEA), with focus on the whole child and the family. It is imperative that psychological support be available, including counseling services. Such services are to be available throughout the child's developmental years, often until adulthood.

Visual Environment: The NAD has always and continues to support and endorse innovative educational programming for deaf children, implanted or not. Such programming should actively support the auditory and speech skills of children in a dynamic and interactive visual environment that utilizes sign language and English.

In closing, the NAD asserts that diversity in communication modes and cultures is our inherent strength, and that mutual respect and cooperation between deaf, hard of hearing, and hearing individuals ultimately benefit us all.

Prepared by the NAD Cochlear Implant Committee
Approved by the NAD Board of Directors
October 6, 2000

Appendix B

Resources for Parenting a Deaf Child

Books

Adams, J. 1997. *You and Your Deaf Child: A Self-Help Guide for Parents of Deaf and Hard of Hearing Children.* Washington, D.C.: Gallaudet University Press.

Luterman, D., and M. Ross. 1991. *When Your Child Is Deaf: A Guide for Parents.* Timonium, Md.: York Press.

Marschark, M. 1997. *Raising and Educating a Deaf Child.* New York: Oxford University Press.

Schwartz, S. 1999. *Choices in Deafness: A Parent's Guide.* Kensington, Md.: Woodbine House.

Organizations

Alexander Graham Bell Association
for the Deaf and Hard of Hearing
3417 Volta Place, N.W.
Washington, D.C. 20007
(202) 337-5220
www.agbell.org

American Society for Deaf Children
P.O. Box 3355
Gettysburg, Penn. 17325
(717) 334-7922
www.deafchildren.org

Beginnings for Deaf Children
P.O. Box 17646
Raleigh, N.C. 27619
(919) 850-2746
www.beginningssvcs.com

John Tracy Clinic
806 West Adams Boulevard
Los Angeles, Calif. 90007
(800) 522-4582
www.jtc.org

National Association of the Deaf
814 Thayer Avenue
Silver Spring, Md. 20910
(301) 587-1788 (V)
(301) 587-1789 (TTY)
www.nad.org

Websites

Advanced Bionics Corporation
www.cochlearimplant.com

Cochlear Corporation
www.cochlear.com

Med El Corporation
www.medel.com

Deafness Research Foundation
www.hearinghealth.net

Alexander Graham Bell Association
for the Deaf and Hard of Hearing
www.agbell.org

Cochlear Implant Association, Inc. (formerly CICI)
www.ciai.org

Self Help for the Hard of Hearing
www.shhh.org

John Tracy Clinic
www.johntracy.org

Oral Deaf Education Website
www.oraldeaf.org

Auditory Verbal International
www.auditory-verbal.org

Appendix C

Published Resources on Cochlear Implants

Books

Christiansen, John, and Irene Leigh. 2002. *Cochlear Implants in Children: Ethics and Choices.* Washington, D.C.: Gallaudet University Press.

Estabrooks, Warren, ed. 1998. *Cochlear Implants for Kids.* Washington, D.C.: A. G. Bell Association.

Nevins, Mary Ellen, and Patricia M. Chute. 1996. *Children with Cochlear Implants in Educational Settings.* San Diego: Singular Publishing.

Niparko, John K., ed. 2000. *Cochlear Implants: Principles and Practices.* Philadelphia: Lippincott, Williams, and Wilkins.

Tye-Murray, Nancy. 1992. *Cochlear Implants and Children: A Handbook for Parents, Teachers, and Speech and Hearing Professionals.* Washington D.C.: A. G. Bell Association.

Tyler, Richard S., ed. 1993. *Cochlear Implants: Audiological Foundations.* San Diego: Singular Publishing.

Waltzman, Susan B., and Noel Cohen. 2000. *Cochlear Implants.* New York: Thieme.

Articles

McDonald Connor, Carol, Sara Hieber, H. Alexander Arts, and Teresa A. Zwolan. 2000. "Speech, Vocabulary, and the Education of Children Using Cochlear Implants: Oral or Total Communication?" *Journal of Speech, Language and Hearing Research* 43(5):1185–204.

Daya, Hamid, Anne Ashley, Claudine Gysin, and Blake C. Papsin. 2000. "Changes in Educational Placement and Speech Perception Ability after Cochlear Implantation in Children." *Journal of Otolaryngology*, 29(4): 224–28.

Knutson, J. F., R. L. Wald, S. L. Ehlers, and R. S. Tyler. 2000. "Psychological Consequences of Pediatric Cochlear Implant Use." *Annals of Otology, Rhinology and Laryngology* 185 (Suppl.): 109–11.

———. 2000. "Psychological Predictors of Pediatric Cochlear Implant Use and Benefit." *Annals of Otology, Rhinology and Laryngology* 185 (Suppl.): 100–3.

McKinley, Ann M., and Steven F. Warren. 2000. "The Effectiveness of Cochlear Implants for Children with Prelingual Deafness." *Journal of Early Intervention*, 23(4): 252–63.

Robbins, Amy M., Mary J. Osberger, Richard T. Miyamoto, and K. S. Kessler. 1994. "Language Development in Young Children with Cochlear Implants." *Advances in Otorhinolaryngology* 50: 160–66.

Samson-Fang, L., M. Simons-McCandless, and C. Shelton. 2000. "Controversies in the Field of Impairment: Early Identification, Educational Methods, and Cochlear Implants." *Infants and Young Children* 12(4): 77–88.

Svirsky, Mario A., R. B. Sloan, M. Caldwell, and Richard T. Miyamoto. 2000. "Speech Intelligibility of Prelingually Deaf Children with Multichannel Cochlear Implants." *Annals of Otology, Rhinology and Laryngology* 185(Suppl.): 123–25.

Wilson, B. 2000. "Strategies for Representing Speech Information with Cochlear Implants." In *Cochlear Implants: Principles and Practices*, ed. John K. Niparko, 129–72. Philadelphia: Lippincott, Williams, and Wilkins.